SHRINK!

How I

EASILY

Lost 40+ lbs in 5 Months

. . . and Kept It Off!

YOU CAN TOO

by Bruce Michaels

Contents

ACKNOWLEDGEMENTS

I'd like to thank the many friends and family members who have contributed to this book's birthing by their encouraging words. Thanks, too, to my editors, Glenn Cook and Gayle Brookbank for their inestimable, generously-given talents.

Additionally, there have been countless individuals in my life for whom I have undying gratitude, and ultimately, we're all influenced by our experiences. Some of those influences have then, by definition, contributed to this book. I hope that I've been at least somewhat successful in conveying that gratitude over the years, and further, declare it here again.

I must also give thanks to Gary Taubes. He doesn't know it, but it was his work that initially prompted me to make a simple, fateful phone call to a long time friend. That call ultimately led me to my other teachers, Drs. Robert Lustig, Richard Bernstein and David Perlmutter. They don't know it either, but their collective wisdom changed my life, and I thank them.

But this book would not have, *could* not have come into existence – indeed, the story at its core, my physical transformation from porky to trim – would not have occurred without the wisdom, guidance, and infinite patience of my dear friend and oftentimes teacher . . . the recipient of that fateful call, Dr. Michael F. Gorczynski. Mike . . . *this one's for you.*

INTRODUCTION

This isn't a textbook, nor is it a compilation of clinical studies. What it is, or at least what I hope it is, is essentially what I tell those friends whom I've not seen for a while when they ask, "Wow, what happened? Where did your belly go?"

Diet successes and failures are common topics across America (and many other places in the world) today, and most often, stories of failure far outnumber those of success. Having participated in many such conversations – originally from the perspective of failure, but now from one of success – I've reached a level of comfort in describing what I learned, what I did, and explaining, despite my non-scientific background, why it worked (and what's at least equally important) why it *continues* to work.

On occasion, if at a gathering of some sort, the topic will arise and I'll find myself answering the question to a roomful of people, informally. This book is intended to retain that sense of informality; were we in a room together, this is what I'd say.

PREFACE

Why did I write this book? Am I qualified? Well, I'm neither a nutritionist nor a dietician, and although I *have* been on TV, I didn't play a doctor. A quick, on-line search or casual glance at your public library or local bookseller's shelves will reveal that many who are credentialed have indeed written books on weight loss; many of them have written several. So, the information's out there, isn't it? I mean, what could I possibly bring to the table? Simply, one unique characteristic: my own story, one with more than a few twists, turns and several frustrating setbacks followed by ultimate and lasting success.

See, even though there are myriad books, plans and diets all purporting to reveal the truth and set us on our way to losing weight, we, the population of the United States (and indeed, much of the industrialized world) instead continue to gain weight, a lot of weight. Despite ever-increasing gym memberships, reality-show challenges and an astonishing number of infomercials hawking incredibly imaginative equipment, we continue to pile on the pounds. We may have won 1944-45's version, but the sad fact is Americans are losing today's Battle of the Bulge. I'm sure you see it wherever you go, as do I . . . in Walmart shopping aisles, lines at airports, school playgrounds and anywhere else your day's travels take you. But it's worse than a just a sizeable percentage of us carrying some extra pounds. "Middle aged spread" has long been thought to be a normal part of lost youth, but the individual whose weight was in excess of 300 or even 400 pounds was rare. Not to be unkind, but that sort of obesity was so rare it was considered worthy of a sideshow. Not anymore; according to a June, 2013 article published in the *US National Library of Medicine,* 15.5 *million* Americans fit the description "morbidly obese."

To put it into numerical context, the Centers for Disease Control reports the average Body Mass Index (BMI) for American men is 28.6; for women it's 28.7. Anything over 25 is considered overweight, with 30 and above considered obese. Nearer to 30 than 25 as a group, we're thus closer to being obese than to merely being overweight. In 2001, a "Newsweek" cover shouted the sad fact that 6 million *kids* are seriously overweight. Despite a dozen years of education, focused attention and "healthier" school diets since then, that number is now close to 20 million, so clearly the problem continues to worsen.

But I digress. Why did I write this book? Because:

Like so many others, I struggled to lose weight, and that struggle lasted years. Now, it's true, I was never obese. In fact, as a kid, I was skinny (when I got a little older and my vocabulary improved I became "svelte"). As an adult, I had a build quite like Barney Fife, although at 5 foot 7, Don Knotts had about 2 inches on me (I briefly considered a career as a jockey). But over time, as I moved from my 30's into my 40's, my waistline started to grow, and as more time passed, it *continued* to grow. Slowly, sure, but grow it did. But for the longest time, I just didn't think it would be much of a problem (famous last words). My history, my truth for so long, was that I could eat an entire box of doughnuts and anything else in sight but still – to my dismay – never gain an ounce. Now, as my waistline gained unwanted inches, I thought I'd just have to, you know, "start paying a bit of attention for a change." No more 6 hot dog-4 beer baseball games. No more 4 hamburger-2 hot dog and lots of potato salad cookouts, and *certainly* no more second and third helpings of coconut cream pie! A modest change . . . pay a bit of attention . . . how hard could it be?

So it was very troubling to discover that, even after I made changes to my diet and ate "normal" portions, my waistline *still* continued to grow. And it continued to expand despite even more changes: exercise, *small* portions (instead of "normal"), less fat consumed, 2%, then 1%, then skim milk, ice cream went from every night to once a week . . . nothing deterred my now seemingly-autonomous waistline from proceeding – to paraphrase a football lineman's stated goal – "to impose its will on me, against my wishes." Physique-wise, I'd gone from Barney Fife to Archie Bunker. I should add that, while I focused on my waistline, inches also piled on to other places. My face, my back, my shoulders, my neck, my butt . . . I went from being wearing boys-sized 16 shirts to having absolutely no hope of that; after I outgrew boys-sized 18 shirts, the men's sized shirts that replaced them fit my frame, but now I couldn't find my hands because the sleeves were too long! I couldn't button my suit coats either; four to five inches gaped from button to buttonhole.

Probably because back in the day, when I couldn't gain an ounce, I never formed the habit of weighing myself, and when I began "expanding" I still didn't weigh myself often. My weight stood at 111 lbs when full-grown in my early 20's, and my waistline was 30 inches. I kept track of my expansion more by my waistline – pants size – than by reading a scale; only occasionally checking my actual weight, I recall being mortified when it neared 140. The highest I ever recall seeing it was 153 (*Gadzooks!*), but that number was so off-putting it was a *long* time before I dared look again. Keep in mind that, for me, 153 pounds represents a nearly 38% gain; if a linebacker, fit at 220 pounds put on that much weight, he'd balloon to over 300 pounds. Likely, too, while I did see 153 once, I probably edged above that before I finally learned how to lose it for good.

But then I did lose it for good. After I did, I'd see people, overweight people, and now knew empathically how they were probably struggling. I'd hear people talking about weight, I'd read newspaper columns, I'd read on-line discussions; we're nearly obsessed with weight loss. I watched a local TV personality endure a pretty strict diet of portion control and once-a-week, live, on-camera sessions at a gym. Having been through the battle, I changed my outlook; my long-held previous view, "Hey, just stop eating so much" changed to, "Wow, I fully understand just how hard it can be."

Career-wise, over the years I've done many things, but one of the several things I currently do is play the organ at baseball games. I'm right out there in the box seats, and for years I've watched individuals – those whom medicos would call "morbidly obese" – move up or down the stairs of the grandstand with great difficulty, and try to fit uncomfortably into their seats.

Having been a stadium organist for over a dozen years, making that observation wasn't a new thing. What *was* new – now being *svelte* again – was my wanting to approach them and say something like, "I know you don't know me, and please forgive me in advance, for even though this may seem rude, I very much don't wish to be. I know you must be unhappy with your weight, I know you must feel your body has betrayed you. Perhaps you feel you got a really unlucky 'weight ticket' in the raffle of life. But even though I'm just a musician, I can help. I learned the secret. No, I'm not the guy who made the discoveries, but because of dumb luck, I recently learned of these things and they *work!*"

Naturally, social mores prevented me from that approach. So with some sadness at being helpless, I'd remain silent and instead think, "If only you knew what I know, if only I could tell you what I've learned." And it was at the ballpark, during a moment like that, when, serendipitously, a couple of thoughts coalesced: "EBooks have revolutionized publishing, truly democratized it," along with, "Wow! That means I *can* share what I've learned."

This is the result.

SHRINK!

UP DOWN UP!

My story of an expanding waistline isn't unique, or even very remarkable. Beginning in my 30's, I found that instead of – as I always had, previously – wishing I could add a few pounds here and there, the pounds added themselves. *Finally!* Except to both my surprise and chagrin, these newly-arrived pounds seemed to have their own idea of where they'd set up housekeeping. Instead of adding a bit of bulk to my chest and shoulders, which would have made for a very nice V-shaped torso, for reasons of their own they thought my waistline more inviting. Oh, and they also brought their friends to my face, neck, back and butt. As I said, that's not so remarkable; in fact, here in America it's probably the norm, but remember, for me this was an entirely new experience.

Well, not to worry; shoot, all my life I ate everything in sight and couldn't gain a pound. Thus, I had only to cut back to "normal" servings and I'd be right back to my youthful waistline. Except, again surprising me, it didn't work out that way. Eating less made no difference; even as I trimmed my food intake I continued to get rounder.

Now, I've always been a voracious reader and my memory was always good. I could readily recall arcane articles on subjects that interested me . . . how radial tires were made . . . the development of the silicon chip . . . how meteorologists contributed to Ike's decision on which day to invade Normandy in 1944 . . . the list is eclectic, as are my interests. Much wispier were any memories of reading about diets and weight loss. Inasmuch as I'd had about as much need for that information as for how to knit a pair of socks, if I *had* read anything, it didn't stick, so now when it would have been useful, I couldn't recall any weight-loss information. So I did some new research, and found the widely accepted premise: Eat more calories than you metabolize and you'll gain weight. Conversely, burn more calories than you consume and you'll lose weight, or, "Calories in versus calories out."

Easy enough, and it made sense. If I put 20 gallons of gas in my car and get 20 miles to the gallon, I'll be able to go 400 miles. The math is irrefutable, and aren't we, in the final analysis, fuel-burning machines? If I only go 300 miles, I'll have some extra fuel in the tank, and transferring the metaphor to a body, that extra fuel is turned into fat. Yep . . . easy to understand, and it should be easy to put into practice.

Of course just as with gas mileage, there might be some variance, some nuance. If I drive with a lead foot, I'll burn more fuel per gallon; if I carry some weight in my backpack or pocket through the day I'll burn more calories. There were further fine-points such as genetics and pre-disposition from a variety of sources, but by and large the differences seemed to be only nuance.

Along the way I got married, and at the wedding, one of my out-of-town guests was one of my best friends in the world, Dr. Michael F. Gorczynski, a family practice physician. Sometime during the weekend, I asked his opinion about weight gain. He was an authority, after all . . . he'd been through med school, his daily work was dealing with the body, its health, diseases, injuries, bio-chemistry, and so I wasn't surprised when he agreed with what I'd read, explaining that except in cases of not-so-common glandular diseases, "calories in versus calories out" was what determined one's weight.[1]

---

[1] Actually, he explained that it's more correctly stated, "Energy of a System = Energy In - Energy Out," but in articles, conversations and interviews it's usually shortened to "Calories in versus calories out."

A few years later I was no longer married (a quick aside: I ardently want to proclaim my ex was and is a wonderful woman, one for whom I have never had anything but wishes for success!). By this time, I did have concern about my waistline, because it continued to grow despite my best efforts to shrink it. I mentioned to my brother what struck me as a great mystery: that, while I used to eat a lot and gain nothing, I'd now reduced my daily intake to not much more than coffee and yogurt in the morning and a hot dog, (*maybe* two) at night, *yet I couldn't stop gaining!* Now, my brother takes pride in going to the gym and keeping fit, so it seemed reasonably logical to get his take. He told me the secret was simple: "Just avoid fat. Hot dogs? Well, *that's* your problem it's all fat!"

Check . . . hot dogs, bad. Whole milk, bad. Ok, let's try and eliminate fat from the diet. Skim milk, low-fat yogurt instead of ice cream, more lettuce and low-fat cottage cheese, no more bacon, skin off the chicken, more fish, less meat and no more sugar in the coffee while I'm at it.

You know what? None of it made a difference. My waistline, too big at 32 inches, went to 33 . . . then 34. *Ok, now this is getting serious!* One of the nuances of the weight loss puzzle is, even at rest, muscle tissue burns more calories than fat tissue. Whatever your weight, if more of your body's mass is made of muscle, you'll burn more calories then were those cells fat cells. That's one of the mantras on which home-exercise equipment is sold. And it *is* true, muscle tissue does burn more. Ok, Bruce . . . eating less food, with nearly zero fat hasn't worked, so . . . ~*sigh*~ . . . we'll add exercise to the equation.

I must disclose here, that as an entertainer, I've for years used a funny line both onstage and in casual conversation with friends whenever it seemed to fit. It is funny (I hope), but for me, it's also largely true: "Exercise? *Exercise?* When I want exercise I *get up* and change the channel!" I'll add that I'm happy to join you for tennis, or dancing, or hoops, or golf, or baseball, or touch football, or whatever. Exercise just for its own sake is what I'd usually avoided.

The funny line notwithstanding, exercise time had arrived. Because it seemed easy to integrate into a daily schedule, I started walking, usually early in the morning. It might have been boring, but I found I could easily overcome the boredom with podcasts. With plenty of variety out there, I could feed my eclectic tastes with a wide array of things that interested me. I got a pedometer and set a goal of two miles a day. Today, I honestly can't recall how long I followed this daily routine; it may have been as few as two months, and likely not longer than four. I stopped for two prime reasons: one, winter arrived (that still strikes me as a fine enough reason to stop). But much more salient: it didn't make even the slightest difference. The waistline (and its back, neck, butt cohorts) continued to grow . . . 35 inches . . . then 36.

Oh, there had been a few times when I seemed to gain the upper hand, most notably the first time I attempted the Atkins Diet. Its central premise: Carbohydrates are sugars. Avoid them and the body will start burning fat. Better still, it wasn't necessary to count calories or restrict portions; eat all the dairy and meat you want as well as non-starchy veggies; just avoid carbs and lose weight.

Wow. Not only did this seem to be a magic bullet, it was a magic bullet I could embrace. Had the magic bullet been a diet consisting of, say, bee stingers and grass clippings, I *might* have tried it, so desperate was I to lose my Archie Bunker shape. But I'm pretty confident that I wouldn't have taken delight in the attempt. But, having grown up with a mother who cooked wonderfully, one who included beef stew, roast chicken and countless other dishes made with meat as part of our daily fare, I'd grown attached to meat as a diet staple. And like every other baby-boomer, I grew up watching westerns. You know, cowboy movies, cowboy TV shows . . . cowboys on horses herding cattle, roping cattle, sitting around campfires roasting cattle. Eating meat had become – how could it be otherwise? – part of my "self."

Let me quickly add: I'm not disapproving of vegetarians. But we've all developed habitual behaviors, deeply entrenched ones. Eating meat and enjoying it is habitual for me. So how could I not give Atkins a try? I don't just mean try it, I mean try it *with enthusiasm!*

I started reading labels and articles just to gain an acquaintance with what had a lot of carbs and what didn't. Corn: out. Pork & beans: out. Broccoli: good stuff. Meat, dairy, eggs, all good. Beer: definitely a no-no (*oh, well*). Potatoes and rice: off the table. Pasta dishes: *Begone, villains!*

It was a little difficult having to forego some things I liked, but after just a couple of weeks, when I noticed positive results it became a lot easier to bear. The size 36 pants that had just about needed to be replaced were getting easy to fasten. I could tighten belts a notch. And after a month and a half or so, I could put a fist into the waistline of those pants; I'd shifted into reverse, and the weight was now steadily coming off. The annoyance of avoiding some of those foods I'd liked evaporated; any slight annoyance was easily countered by the success I was seeing. After about 3 or 4 months, I was at a "suitable" place. My older clothes fit; I wasn't any longer embarrassed by my profile. This was like winning the Super Bowl . . . *I'm going to Disneyland!*

After declaring victory, I modified my diet. "Ok, now that I'm finally 'down,' I'll eat more carefully, and monitor my weight" (or, more accurately, my waistline). "Surely, I can now have the occasional beer or modestly-sized plate of spaghetti."

Or so I thought. Yes, I'd avoided carbs and lost weight, but I still really didn't understand why it worked. Something about "ketosis," I think; yeah, that was it, ketosis. Maybe.

Honestly, though, I really didn't care why. It was a blissful ignorance, and one not very dissimilar from a driver who turns the ignition switch and drives off without ever understanding that gasoline is pumped from the tank to the engine, is vaporized, compressed and then combusts with enough explosive force to turn a crankshaft.

But because I didn't understand even an iota of the bio-chemistry involved, I was pretty much doomed to another round of weight-gain. In all the books, all the discussions, in all the interviews, the phenomenon of yo-yoing weight is well documented, and I was about to discover its ugly reality. I resumed a "normal" diet, albeit it one without large portions, without seconds and very modest allowances for only an occasional dessert. And yet, slowly, almost imperceptibly, the weight started to return.

A couple years, maybe three elapsed, and I had to quite unhappily confront the fact that I again needed unpack the larger pants.

"Well," I thought, "I did it before, I'll just do Atkins again. And when done, I'll be even *more* severe with my 'normal' diet . . . hell's bells, I may even return to exercise!"

I recall clearly that I began on a Monday morning. "Wow! I don't remember it being *this* difficult!" And it *was* more difficult this time. The first time, my appetite was pretty happy to accept large quantities of meat, fish and cheese in place of those specifically *verboten* foods (corn, bread, pasta, beer, etc.), but this go-round, even after eating good-sized portions of the allowable foods, I felt . . .

Y'know, it's actually very difficult to describe *what* I felt. It certainly wasn't hunger; I'd eat until quite full. The word I'll use is "unsatisfied," but that doesn't exactly convey what I felt, either. But "unsatisfied" was only for the first two days. By Wednesday that week, "unsatisfied" had morphed into something else, a monstrous craving so powerful I believe it was like being in the middle of a hot desert for days without water. I ate several meals, I ate lots of food, but still something inside craved. Craved? *Lusted* is more like it!

By Thursday evening I was beyond miserable. I hadn't had sugar in my coffee, I hadn't had ice cream, but inside, it felt as though every cell in my body was screaming, "I WANT A POTATO!!!!" (Which was weird, because – even though as an adult I grew to appreciate a fine baked potato or well-flavored mashed potatoes – as a I kid I tended to avoid them (except, of course, french fries)). Of everything out there I might crave . . . a potato? Weird.

Well, Thursday night I crumpled. I had better never become a prisoner of war or a spy with secrets, because if the enemy reads this book, they'll know I'll give up PIN numbers, passwords, nuclear secrets, my first-born (*ha-ha, fooled them, I've got no kids!*); I'll give up *anything* for a potato. And so it was that Thursday night I had something with starch in it. I don't now remember what I ate that night, but I do remember the extreme bliss I felt as those carbs hit my innards and washed out into my bloodstream. Maybe not quite orgasmic, perhaps, but . . . well, maybe it was orgasmic, after all. It certainly was blissful!

The next little "chapter" in this ongoing battle of the bulge will be very short, but before I give you the details, I want to explain why I can't provide an exact timeline for some of these events. I can't because I was living my life: working, playing, reading, eating . . . you know, *living* . . . and while I was personally frustrated by my failures, I wasn't documenting any of this. I've never kept a diary, so I can only plumb my memory for the times and sequences. The first use of Atkins (the successful one) was perhaps in 2003 or 2004. The 2nd attempt, the one that lasted four days took place around 2007. At the time of that 2nd attempt, I hadn't yet re-swollen to the size 36 pants, so I didn't feel desperate. Yes, there had again been expansion, so I again attempted Atkins. Perhaps it was simply the lack of desperation that sufficiently weakened my determination so that four days' worth was all the willpower I could muster.

But by around 2010, I was again up to size 36. Although I clearly recalled my failure with "Atkins Part II," I was pretty confident that this time, given the "emergency" – SIZE 36! – I could surely summon the strength of character with which I'd succeeded the first time. I braced myself and began. I knew it would be difficult, but hey, I could do it. Unlike "Atkins Part II," this time more was riding on it . . . my self-esteem, potential income (I'm a performer), expenses (I didn't have bigger than 36 pants, nor were my suits fitting; if I needed bigger suits, a new wardrobe wasn't likely fall from the sky). So, fully steeled and resolute, I began. This time I have no memory – clear or otherwise – on which day of the week I began. But I can tell you exactly the day it ended, for that memory is clear; it was the *same day.*

Yes, sadly . . . despite the confidence, the bracing, the foreknowledge that it would be difficult, despite the various motivating factors, by the *evening* of Day One, none of it mattered. Again as desperate as the thirsty man in the desert, I was hearing my cells shouting, "I WANT A POTATO!" Come to think of it, I may have actually shouted out loud, "DAMN IT, I *NEED* A POTATO!" Feeling guilty, but altogether helpless I dove into the carbs.

I told you the telling of this 3rd attempt would be brief.

2. NOW WHAT DO I DO?

This turn of events had me pretty-well bombed out. Most of my life I'd been skinny - I mean *svelte* – and could look good in a well-tailored suit. It was disconcerting when I started to gain weight, but despite the ups and downs, I always internally held the confidence that I'd – somehow – be able to regain a trim waist. After some initial failures, I'd found success with my first go around with Atkins and thought I had the secret. I attributed the second attempt's failure to merely not being sufficiently motivated; I wasn't, after all, at "the limit."

But there was no disguising this latest failure. Enormously motivated, and I still couldn't make it even twenty four hours? I now considered any number of other solutions, including doctor-prescribed diet pills, liposuction (fat cells literally sucked out of the body), gastric bypass surgery and extreme fasting. I knew the first three were weren't feasible; diet pills can produce pretty severe side effects, and while my waistline and double chin were mortifying to me, I wasn't anywhere near the kind of obesity that would persuade a physician to either prescribe pills or perform the medical procedures (nor could I have afforded the latter).

It seemed that I'd just have to eat less and cut more calories from my diet . . . maybe fast a couple days a week, even more if need be. I did; it wasn't much fun, but worse, I didn't lose weight. I did, though, at least largely succeed in preventing additional inches. As I'd mentioned previously, I'd never been one to get on a scale often. When I was skinny, it was depressing, when I was svelte it was all good so why bother? And when I was gaining weight, I already knew I was putting it on; getting on a scale only seemed a way to become further depressed about it.

I do recall the highest number the scale revealed to me, though I can't specify when that last reading took place. My best guess is that it was late 2010 or early 2011, but having seen it spin to 153, I wasn't in a hurry to again get more bad news. Over time, I may have drifted up or down from that by a couple/three pounds, but as I said, my limited food intake had at least pretty well stabilized my enlarging body.

Stabilized or not, I still wanted my old body back; I know, I know, that's a desire shared by millions. That shared desire, of course, spawns countless books, magazine articles and tabloid headlines: *Get Your*

Body Beach-Ready in Six Weeks! and the like. I'd occasionally peruse one of those articles, or watch someone promoting something on TV, and while some of these things seemed truly plucked out of fantasy – *Eat This One Berry & Lose 10 lbs a Week!* – I didn't see any that were both science-based and differing from the "Count calories and exercise" mantra. Big deal; I'd already found *that* didn't work, at least for me.

But sometime in the spring of 2011 – my timeline now definitely becomes more focused – I encountered an interview with Gary Taubes. His recent book, "*Why We Get Fat: And What to Do About It*" had just been published a few months earlier. Busy with other tasks, I paid only slight attention, just enough to glean that its premise was "carbs are bad."

"Oh, ok," I thought, "it's like Atkins." Having quite spectacularly failed with Atkins twice and with my attention focused on other projects, I saw no reason to delve any deeper at the time.

It was later that summer, still struggling to discover a way back to my svelte self, but now with time enough to revisit the issue when I more closely studied what Taubes had to say. The first thing I discovered was he wasn't new to the subject, but in fact had previously published *"Good Calories, Bad Calories,"* a book similar in theme, but more technically oriented, more directed to the scientific community. Indeed, that's what Taubes is, a science writer. With a BS from Harvard in applied physics, a Master's in aerospace engineering from Stanford and a Master's in journalism from Columbia, he's obviously a smart guy. In his book, he points out that the conventional wisdom of *calories in vs. calories out* is a relatively recent invention. Moreover, he argues that several studies have been ignored, even though they *refute* calories in vs. calories out. Still, I was skeptical; from the cursory understanding I had, he seemed to be making the case against carbs and sugars, and I'd had two successive failures going that route.

Intrigued though, and still hoping to find some avenue to success, I called my friend, Dr. Michael F. Gorczynski. He's one of my very closest friends, and over the years we'd spoken of just about everything imaginable: Family, politics, sports and of course, matters of health. I've always known I was fortunate; if I, or a family member had a procedure, a symptom or a prescription, I could always pick up the phone and ask something like, "Hey, Mike . . . my mom's been told by her doctor that . . . what does that mean in English?" And he'd explain it in a way so understandable I could then explain it to someone else in a way that *they* would understand.

So (take note of the date), in either very late July or very early August of 2011, I called. "I've been hearing and reading about a book that's getting some buzz called 'Why We Get Fat,' by Gary Taubes. Are you familiar with it, have you read it?"

Before I tell of his reply, I want to tell you a little about him, even at the risk of causing him to blush a bit. Not only is he a physician and thus obviously well-learned about human biology, he's a critical thinker, willing to seek answers on his own and form his own opinions. Over the years, I'd discovered that his critical thinking had on occasion led him away from simple, reflexive acceptance of conventional wisdom. Yes, he's mainstream, but yes, too, he forms conclusions by more than simply staying abreast of the latest study's summary; he reads the whole thing. That's the background with which I want to frame the conversation of that summer day in 2011.

"Hey, Mike . . . have you heard about or read this book by Gary Taubes?"

"No, I haven't read it. But I'm familiar with it, and what it suggests."

It was the first of several conversations I'd have with him on the subject over several months, and with each conversation, he'd teach me a bit more and I'd gain a little better understanding of what drives weight gain. During that call, he also recommended I watch a lecture on youtube called, "Sugar: The Bitter Truth," presented by Dr. Robert Lustig.

At the conversation's end, I didn't know if any of this would turn out to be useful. But I thought I'd at least take a closer look at the book and probably watch the video, all in the hope of finding the missing "milk-carton person" most dear to me: my svelte self.

3. SYNCHRONICITY

I've said I love a wide variety of information, and I love it whether I find it in print, in film, on-line, broadcasts or podcasts. My interests are varied, but not infinite; I was fascinated to read Benjamin Franklin's essay about farting (of all things!), I was surprised to learn that Bob Dylan – *many* years ago – auditioned to play piano in Bobby Vee's backup band, I was riveted by a film documenting the evolution of the forward pass in football, but I really could not care any less about, say, the origins of weaving.

The Peoples Pharmacy is a radio program that airs on many NPR stations. It's a program that I often listen to as it airs, but if I miss it, I check the "recent shows" listing at their website, www.peoplespharmacy.com. Depending on the topic, I may or may not elect to listen or download the podcast. The show's co-hosts, Joe & Terry Graedon, discuss health news, then usually focus on a specific topic, interviewing guests whose expertise fits that topic. Often the guest is an author.

On the morning of Saturday, August 5, 2011 – note, this is just a few days after my conversation with Dr. Mike – their guest was Gary Taubes. The topic was indeed his recent book, "Why We Get Fat: and What to Do About It." Synchronicity can be defined as "a coincidence of events that seem to be meaningfully related." Well, this surely fit that!

Taubes' time on the show was roughly forty five minutes; in that brief time, it would have been impossible for him to explain everything he wrote in his book. But I learned that morning that, if nothing else, his conclusions were based on his reviewing many weight-loss studies, a reading of the researchers' own words, and a historical, long view of how we came to believe counting calories was the way to control one's weight.

He held my attention, and I determined to get his book; following the show, I immediately checked with the local library . . . they had it, it was available and I picked it up the same day. I'd finished it by the end of the weekend, and was now seriously interested in learning more. Though I'm a world-class procrastinator, there *are* times when I can get going!

Motivated now, I went on-line to youtube to find the video Dr. Mike recommended: Dr. Robert Lustig's "Sugar: The Bitter Truth." Despite its length of an hour and a half, I found it compelling. I admit my mind wandered just a little bit during the few minutes he explains some bio-chemistry in deeper medical terms than I understand, but that's a small part of the whole. I understood most of it, and it's easy to watch, as he's an engaging, entertaining speaker.

The points he makes in the presentation aren't *exactly* the same as Taubes', but their trajectories use evidence . . . *data*. . . to reach largely the same conclusions. And while I may not have understood all the bio-chemistry Dr. Lustig explained, I understood the points well enough to be able to take action. (Dr. Lustig also takes particular aim at what's become nearly unavoidable in the American diet: high fructose corn syrup, a subject we'll return to later.)

By sometime in mid-August – maybe it was nearer Labor Day – I was ready to begin. I made some pretty fundamental changes to what I would eat and drink and braced myself for what I thought might be a difficult experience. But here's what's most interesting: while the changes *were* fundamental, they were *easy* when compared to what I'd experienced in the past. No innards screaming, no self-identification with Frank Sinatra's portrayal of "The Man With the Golden Arm."

(For those who don't recall that film, Sinatra played a heroin addict who'd been clean, but again succumbs to temptation.   Needing a fix, his on-screen agony is riveting;   it resulted in an Oscar nomination for Sinatra. It's not a stretch to say "Atkins Part III" made me feel the same way.)

But this time there was no agony for me, none. In fact, the single, *most* difficult change was not sweetening my morning coffee. I used to be nearly unwavering in my coffee consumption: two cups (ok, mugs, you know, *real world* cups) in the morning, and rarely would I have any more the rest of the day. But those two cups . . . I cherished them. They were part of my morning ritual, part of waking up: coffee with the news, the newspapers, the funnies and word puzzles. On weekends I'd up the ante and enjoy it even more: I'd use *expensive* coffee! (My experience has been, if I used really good coffee every morning, its "special-ness" dissipated, and it became "the norm," i.e., ordinary. Ordinary coffee during the weekdays meant I could more completely savor the richness of the good stuff on weekends.)

For me, that cherished coffee included cream and sugar, so foregoing sugar was indeed a sacrifice; I was giving up one of life's simple pleasures, and to this day, it's what I miss most. But "sacrifice" is a relative term. I'm not Abraham on Mount Moriah with Isaac. I'm not struggling with severe cravings . . . I'm not *suffering!* My "sacrifice" of drinking unsweetened coffee is an *inconvenience*, nothing more.

Now, if I had followed this new eating regimen for several months *without* result, I'm pretty sure I'd have said, "The hell with it, why have even the inconvenience if it makes no difference" and returned to sweetening my coffee. Months did pass, but the results weren't merely noticeable, they were astonishingly dramatic! Making it all so much "sweeter" (I hope you'll forgive the irresistible pun) was that the "inconvenience" of unsweetened coffee remained the hardest, most trying element of my new way of eating! That's it? That's the worst thing? That's the cost of pounds *falling* off? *Excellent!*

So, a couple months had passed, I was feeling pretty good about this stuff when synchronicity struck again. Near the end of November (still 2011), on another episode of "The Peoples Pharmacy," who was the guest? Dr. Robert Lustig! As I remember it, I didn't catch the show live, but instead discovered at the show's website that he'd been the guest, and this was actually fortuitous. Not often, but neither rarely, the Peoples Pharmacy website will provide a podcast of the show as it aired *and* a longer interview, i.e., the full interview before it was edited and shortened to fit into the hour-long program.   This was one of those occasions, and I downloaded the extended interview.

This was getting better all the time.   Naturally, he iterated some of the same points he'd made in his youtube presentation, but he also made many new ones (new to me, anyway).   I gained a much better understanding of *why* what I was doing was working so well, and my enthusiasm to continue this effective way of eating elevated even more.

As I've said, I didn't begin this as a lab rat, so I didn't set out to keep vital statistics and dates and results; I only wanted to lose weight.   Now recall, I'm an entertainer.   In February, 2011, while still in my "fat body," I performed my one-man show, "Dinner With the Rat Pack (and more!)" and, fortunately, as it turns out, I have some video footage of that show.   One year later, around Valentine's Day 2012, I performed it again at the same place.   I may not have perfect documentation, but these single-frame captures from the videos provide a stark comparison.   Remember, I'd only been at this new way of eating for about five months at the time of the second Valentine's show. These are video frames, so the quality isn't the best, but the difference is clear.

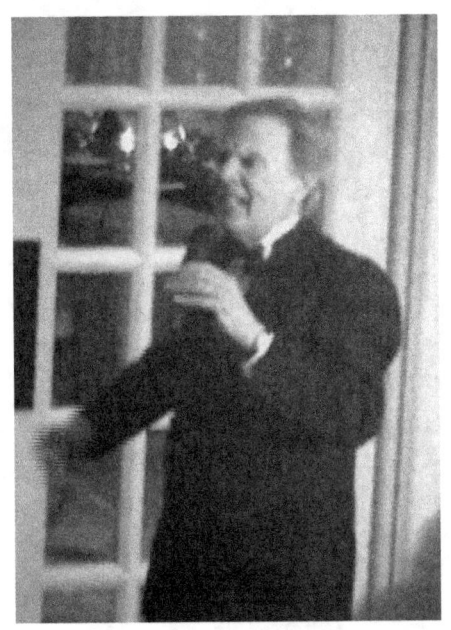

2011

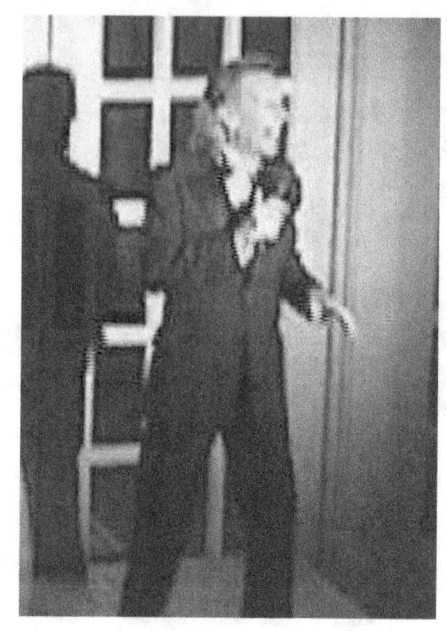

2012

Since I wasn't keeping meticulous records I can only estimate, but at the time of the 2011 show, I'd already experienced my pitiful, second failure on Atkins; my pants size would have been 36 (but needing to be bigger), and my weight was somewhere around 153 pounds. February, 2012, *only five months after I changed eating habits*, my waist size was around 31 (actually a bit under . . . size 31 *required* a belt!) and my weight was likely between 111 and 115. And I was neither hungry nor screaming "Potato!"

I need to again underscore that this "changed eating" wasn't hard to do. It does work, but news that it works isn't by itself important to you. If I could have summoned the will power to just stop eating, or, say, have chicken broth once a day, with mushrooms once a week (or eaten bee stingers and grass clippings), it's likely I would have lost weight and inches. But it's equally likely you'd not be interested in learning about it. In other words, I might have proved that near-starvation "works," but if it's not a reasonable plan, it wouldn't be worth your time to read about it (ok, here I'm *assuming* you wouldn't be interested in a diet of bee stingers and grass clippings). POWs often lose weight in just this way – starvation – but it's not much of a plan. Even if you could summon the enormous will power it would require, once you hit your target weight, you'd stop starving yourself, and the pounds would pile back on.

No, I say again, what makes this experience so extraordinary is that not only does eating this way work, but that it's pretty easy to follow, long term. It's now over two years since the 2012 Valentine's show, and the weight remains off. Earlier, I wrote of the Body Mass Index: To iterate, below 18.5 is considered underweight, 18.5 to 24.9 is considered normal, 25.0 to 29.9 is overweight and 30 and above is considered obese. Although I can only estimate what it was in the summer of 2011 – best guess is approaching 27 – I know it today: my BMI is 18.8. (Gee, it's a good thing for beer, which I do allow myself; without it, I might slip into "underweight!")

So, just a few months into this and thrilled by the startlingly wonderful success, I started talking about it. I also kept seeking more information, the better to bolster what I was telling friends and family. I also spoke frequently with Dr. Mike to better understand what I was learning. There were many sources, but podcasts proved to be a rich vein I continued to mine.

DR. RICHARD BERNSTEIN

In July, 2012, "The Peoples Pharmacy" had Dr. Richard Bernstein as a guest. He's an M.D. who specializes in treating diabetes and who's authored several books on the disease's causes and treatments. Physicians treating diabetes isn't news, but his story comes from a personal perspective: he himself became diabetic at age 12. Though following his physicians' advice through adolescence and adulthood, he, as happens to many diabetics, suffered many devastating health problems including heart damage and kidney disease.

In 1969 he saw an ad for the first blood glucose meter, but it was only available to physicians and hospitals. As an engineer he couldn't purchase it; however, his physician-wife could. Using it, he closely monitored his own blood sugar levels, and discovered that carbs spiked his blood sugar. Acting on his own, while continuing to self-test, he adjusted his carbohydrate consumption and his insulin doses accordingly, with excellent results, including better health. This was a major breakthrough, but despite his success, when he tried to publish his findings, the medical community showed little interest; after all, *he was an engineer, not a health practitioner!*

As he put it, "I couldn't beat 'em, so I had to join 'em." He returned to school, became an M.D., and not only opened his practice to treat diabetes, but is recognized as the inventor of home blood-glucose monitoring. His findings vis a vis carbs and sugars dovetail with those of Gary Taubes and Dr. Robert Lustig: carbohydrates – sugars, all – are potentially poisonous, and many of his patients, following his recommendations, have returned to normal health, i.e., they have normal blood sugar *without the use of insulin!* That podcast, from July 2012, is available at "The Peoples Pharmacy" website; the URL will appear in the appendix.

BACK ONCE AGAIN . . . DR. LUSTIG

Dr. Lustig continues to spread the word. You can readily find his "Bitter Truth" lecture on youtube, but if you do a search for him there now, you'll find he's become a rock star! He appears on *many* videos, as a speaker, as a member of a panel at a forum on nutrition, in an excerpt from "Good Morning America." There's a new lecture, too; in the summer of 2013, he presented "Fat Chance: Fructose 2.0," which is basically a follow-up to "Bitter Truth."

In 2012 he wrote a new book, "Fat Chance: Beating The Odds Against Sugar, Processed Food, Obesity, and Disease." During the book's promotional tour, he appeared on several programs, including NPR's "The Diane Rehm Show" in January, 2013. Yep . . . another podcast, and he was as fascinating as ever.

Near that show's end, Dr. Lustig revealed some frustration. Responding to caller (a nutritionist who reiterated the still-conventional wisdom that "a calorie is a calorie"), his voice was measured, but one could hear in his voice his frustration. My guess is it stemmed from the fact that for years now, he (and others, some listed through this book) has for years been trying to get out the word: *We not only face an obesity epidemic which in turn leads to many other deadly health threats, but what's causing the epidemic is plain to see.* Yet here he was, facing another health professional who refused to accept the evidence he so passionately believes is obvious.

He refuted her position by listing a few specific examples which proved, at least to my satisfaction, a calorie is *not* a calorie. I found it interesting that the nutritionist later posted a youtube video of her own in which she defended her belief and ended with the dramatically spoken words, "A calorie *is* a calorie."

Take that!

Ok, two opposite viewpoints, and I haven't the credentials enabling me to get funding to initiate my own formal research study of the issue. But in my opinion, during his rebuttal he cited several facts clearly showing the fallacy of "a calorie is a calorie." But debate points aside, I think it far more telling that when I followed *his* advice – as opposed to when I tried to follow the recommendations she and the majority still advocate – the weight just fell off my body. So, credentialed or not . . . I'm going with him.

DR. DAVID PERMUTTER

The most recent podcast I found on this topic aired in December, 2013 (as I write this, that was just months ago). Again it was "The Peoples Pharmacy" and the guest was Dr. David Perlmutter, a neurologist who'd recently written a book called "Grain Brain: The Surprising Truth About Wheat, Carbs and Sugar – Your Brain's Silent Killers." He takes carbs to task for a different reason, citing their effects on the brain. He argues that avoiding carbs promotes a healthy brain and helps avoid depression, ADHD, Alzheimer's and dementia.

More recently, during fundraisers in March, 2014, Dr. Perlmutter appeared on many PBS stations across the country during their Spring Fund drive; the program: "BRAINCHANGE."

I've listened to these podcasts several times; I've read many of the books, and believe I've got it pretty well boiled down to a "layman's essence." In the next chapter I'm going to tell you what I make of all this in what I hope is clear language. And in the final chapter I'll tell you what I did; you already know the result. This is what I tell my friends in conversation when the topic arises.

4. MYTHOLOGY 101

So here we are, at the good stuff. After all the reading, listening and questioning, this chapter is intended to boil down all that information into what I hope is a condensation more easily understood by someone like me: a person of reasonable intelligence without a science or medical background. While I can't explain in exacting detail the metabolic processes, I can explain what I understand to be true and why. In the previous chapters I told my story, the gaining and losing weight, gaining it back but *failing* to lose it again. I also told how these insights came to me in stages, through several different sources and messengers. Once I achieved that insight, I was able to put into practice what I learned, and it worked far better and far more easily than I'd ever dreamed possible.

Before you put it in practice, I'd suggest you read some or all of the books I mention; watch the videos and listen to the podcasts. In the appendix I list the websites and books I'm writing about, but as I continue to discover, there are many others out there saying the same things. The podcasts may require a modest purchase price to download, but all this information is readily available. It's not *my* health or weight you're responsible for, it's yours. Do your research; discover the facts to *your* satisfaction.

And one last point, mandated by the legal department: at some point you will or will not elect to adopt this plan, but this isn't a medical book. If it sounds good to you and you want to try it yourself, you should check with your own doctor first. He or she may say, "Hey, that's great, I've been seeing more and more of this lately." Or, he/she may disagree with what I suggest, and perhaps even recoil in horror! That shouldn't surprise; while this information is steadily gaining traction, it hasn't yet reached the tipping point. If your physician is of the latter group, show him this information, as presented in the podcasts, books and videos.

In my opinion, the tipping point will be reached sooner rather than later. Today's "conventional wisdom" on weight loss every day loses believers, and I can't help but think it will inevitably go the way of other once-believed, but now discredited "truths," such as *powered flight will never be possible.*

Personally, I think this news is like the coming of spring; winter has the upper hand, cold days far outnumber the warm. But after warm days make their initial appearance, they occur with greater frequency, they then gain equality and inevitably overtake the cold days, ultimately vanquishing them to memory. If your physician isn't familiar with this information and doubts its truth, share this info and point to the books, vids and podcasts. *My* credentials won't impress, but the authorities' I cite will, and my guess is you'll get a big thank you!

What I find remarkable about this obesity epidemic is that it's exploded *despite* unprecedented investment in fitness. President Kennedy's administration began an emphasis on fitness, but that was only a baby step compared to the focus today. We see gyms just blocks away from each other, outnumbering by far the "full-service" gas stations that were once ubiquitous. Every supermarket has shelves of "healthy" (usually meaning low-fat) foods and there are even chain supermarkets devoted *exclusively* to whole and organic foods. Home exercise equipment can be bought in stores, on-line, through magazine ads and on TV shopping networks. Institutions of higher learning offer "Personal Trainer" as a career choice! Richard Simmons pioneered video tapes in which he led us through exercise to music; today there are many more exercise gurus following in his footsteps (although today they're on DVD). There are any number of diet plans you can subscribe to and some will even send food directly to your home. Talk about convenience! No thinking caps needed, you don't have to count calories or portions, you don't have to consider what's healthy, you don't have to plan; you only have to subscriber and these "healthy meals will reduce your weight." You can even buy stuff you sprinkle on your food that causes you to eat less.

(Uhm . . . y'know, there are any number of things you could get for free that would accomplish the exact same thing, but we won't go there . . .)

Radio, TV, news magazines, newspapers, tabloids all regularly run stories on how to lose weight. Those stories wouldn't run so frequently if we weren't interested, but we *are* interested, so those stories always capture large audiences.

And yet, despite all of this . . . we have an obesity epidemic that is at once both catastrophic and getting worse. By that, I don't mean we've become a nation whose middle-aged population all have "spare tires;" I mean, instead, our population includes many *grossly* overweight individuals, and in all age groups! How can these two facts co-exist? How can we pay enormous attention to weight and fitness, have so many ways to shed pounds, and *still be losing the battle?*

In a word: Myths.

What we've been told for several decades – these myths – have proved to be untrue. Understand, I'm not saying they were made up just for fun, or that they were spun out of whole cloth with some kind of ulterior motive designed to make us fat.

(Ok, anything's possible, I suppose, but I don't believe that. Nor do I believe Elvis is alive and chilling out in Ecuador.)

Instead, what I believe happened is the scientific community made an honest mistake in analyzing some evidence. It certainly wasn't the first time, and it won't be the last. But because it seemed so right intuitively, it was hard to dismiss, even after further examination didn't corroborate those mistaken beliefs. *Look at the ground; the earth is flat, anyone can see that!* Well, of course, we now know it's not flat, but the old belief gave ground grudgingly before the truth was finally accepted.

Or this: *"Peyton Manning and the 2013 Denver Broncos proved to be the most prolific scoring machine the NFL has ever seen. Of course they'll win the Super Bowl."*

Today, post 2014's Super Bowl, a devoted Broncos fan, an ardent believer of that pre-game prediction might now say something like, *"Yes, I know, the Broncos lost. But it was just one game...a fluke! The Broncos would win next time!* It's human nature to hold fast to those things we believe, and the scientific community – human beings, all – is no different. So, along with a comment or two, here are the myths. We'll then look at each in more detail.

MYTH NUMBER ONE: MAINTAINING WEIGHT MEANS BALANCING CALORIES IN WITH CALORIES OUT

As I'd written earlier in this book, I, too, thought this is self-evident; how could it *not* be true? I mean, it's just simple math, right? As we'll see, not exactly.

MYTH NUMBER TWO: EXERCISE MORE AND EAT LESS . . . THAT'S HOW TO LOSE WEIGHT

This is a widespread belief, I know. It's obviously intuitive, and is the mirror to Myth Number One. But it just isn't a very effective weight-loss strategy.

MYTH NUMBER THREE: FAT IS BAD FOR YOU, IT'S THE ULTIMATE ENEMY

Turns out, this is also false, but with a qualifier: Some fats *are* bad for you; but others are not only not bad, they're healthy, they're absolutely essential to good health.

MYTH NUMBER FOUR: CHOLES- TEROL IS BAD AND CAUSES HEART DISEASE

Yes, there are qualifiers here, too, and you may already be aware that there are "good cholesterols" and "bad cholesterols." But there's *far* more to it than that.

MYTH NUMBER FIVE: A HEALTHY DIET IS REPRESENTED BY THE USDA'S FOOD PYRAMID

The USDA food pyramid was first introduced in 1992, and even before the pyramid, the USDA has published nutritional guidelines. As a concept – providing information that consumers can use to make informed decisions about what to eat – it's a fine idea. The problem is the advice hasn't been consistent. We all joke that the guidelines change: "First they tell us "XXXX" is good. Then it's bad. Now it's good again. Do they know *anything?*"

Who could blame you for becoming jaded? We hear of studies and their results; new guidelines are issued. Then a few years later those guidelines are contradicted by newer studies. Of course when it comes from scientists, our nature is to embrace new info. After all, scientists know more than they ever did before, we have better understanding, we have atomic microscopes and computer-modeling . . . don't we? Yes, we do. But let me posit this thought: the very fact that the pyramid has been modified several times proves its fallibility.

Wow! So these are all myths? Myths!?!? Surely not! These are the very lynchpins of contemporary nutrition wisdom. Aren't they?

The answer is, yes, they are, but my opinion – and the opinion of many others – is they'll remain lynchpins for only for a little while longer. They've had their run, the evidence doesn't support them and the tide is indeed turning; to see why, let's now examine these myths one at a time.

MYTH NUMBER ONE: MAINTAINING WEIGHT MEANS BALANCING CALORIES IN WITH CALORIES OUT

This is, for me, the most beguiling myth of them all. Its symmetry is exquisite, even poetic. Earlier, I used the metaphor of my car. If I fill the tank and drive, I can: a) drive until my fuel is exhausted; b) stop when I'm nearly out of fuel and put more in the tank; c) drive some distance and stop with some gas left in the tank. In option "c)" the gas left in the tank is thus excess fuel, and for this metaphor, represents fat. Who doesn't get that? Don't we humans, in fact all life, burn and replenish fuel?

But under scrutiny, the metaphor doesn't hold up. The simple math assumes certain things. In most discussions and examples, the average person is said to require about 2000 calories a day. In reality, much depends on your personal metabolism, how active and old you are, your genetics, how much you weigh and even what you've eaten *throughout* your life. A 200 pounder carries 200 pounds through the day's activities, while a 100 pounder is obviously carrying half that load. But for discussion's sake, we can use 2000 calories; it's as good a baseline as any.

The first flawed assumption is that a calorie is a calorie, but that's only true while it's outside the body; it's not true once ingested. Let's say you have a standard, 12 oz. can of Coke; if you drink it you'll have consumed 140 calories. But what if, instead of a Coke, you eat almonds, exactly 140 calories worth of almonds. An equal number of calories should mean equal results, right?

Ah, but the almonds have fiber, a good deal of fiber, and as a result, once consumed those 140 calories are handled very differently by the body. Dr. Lustig describes in some detail how fiber causes those differences in his books, on the youtube seminar, and during his radio appearances. After reading, watching and listening to them, here's my own, non-medical understanding of fiber's benefits:

One, it slows the absorption of the calories, which means they don't get into your bloodstream as quickly. That's good, because a spike in blood sugar is bad (as we'll see in more detail shortly).

Two, not only is the absorption slower, the fiber *accelerates* the transport of the almonds through your

G.I. tract; this means some of those calories *never get absorbed as fuel by the body at all!* Why? Because roughly 19% of the almonds' 140 calories are consumed by *bacteria* in the gut. This is fundamental to understanding why simple calorie-counting can't work, because *what* you eat to get those calories enormously influences how many your body keeps for itself; that's far more important than just knowing how many calories are in a particular food.

Let's go a step further, and use an example as explained by Dr. Perlmutter. Would you have a standard, 12 oz. can of Coke for breakfast? (I'm assuming you're not a fifteen year old boy, who might smile widely and answer, "Dude! Awesome!") Everybody knows the Coke (or any other non-artificially sweetened soft drink) has what are known as "empty calories," i.e., they contain calories, but no nutrition. We all agree. But would you have 12 oz. of orange juice for breakfast? Easy answer . . . fifteen year old boy or not, many of us, most of us probably, would say yes to that. Tastes good, it's natural, it's fruit, for heaven's sake; of course it's good!

Well, it does have Vitamin C as well as potassium and other good things, so unlike the Coke there is some nutrition. But here's the catch: the OJ doesn't have fiber. Twelve ounces of orange juice has 34 grams of carbohydrates (sugars) compared to Coke's 36 grams; 34 to 36? Geez, hardly any difference. A twelve ounce glass of orange juice has the equivalent of nine – count 'em, **nine!** – teaspoons of sugar in it! Without the fiber, those nine teaspoons worth of sugars get absorbed into the bloodstream just as rapidly as they would from Coke.

I think that's pretty simple to understand, but there's an even more sinister element involved in this, and that's the role the sugar itself plays in this little drama. Its role can't be overstated, and unfortunately, the news is bad. Now, keep in mind, when I use the word sugar, I'm not referring only to the sweet white stuff I now leave out of my coffee, I'm referring to all sugars. All carbohydrates, complex or not, become sugar once in the body. I know, we all grew up with certain traditional, *yummy* foods: lavish, multi-tiered wedding cakes, cotton candy or funnel cakes at the fair, Halloween candy, Christmas cookies, ice cream cones, coconut-cream pie and countless other treats that are all but irresistible. Ok, we know those things are laden with sugar, but what about rice? Matzo ball soup? Yes. And yes, too, to cornbread (plain corn, in fact, and plain bread, too), pretzels, hot dog buns, pinto beans, potato chips (and plain old potatoes, for that matter). Lots of starch in all of those, and once in the body, they're all sugars.

"Okay, I know, sugar is fattening. But really, if I have just a bit now and again, what's the harm?"

The truth is, a little now and then probably won't cause much harm, and you must have some sugar in your bloodstream. But depending on how much you ingest, and how quickly it gets into the bloodstream, sugar has toxic effects. Yes, you read it correctly; sugar can be a toxin, and when it's ingested, the body works pretty quickly to lower its concentration in the bloodstream. When there's constantly too much sugar in the blood, bad things can occur, including blindness, kidney failure and a host of other maladies.

Remember, sugar in small amounts is vital, our brains can't function without it. In nature, especially in the forms our ancestors ate (whole fruits, for example) foods provided the necessary amounts, but also had the added benefit of arriving in packages laden with fiber. (It's probably worth noting, too, that the fruits and other carb products our ancestors ate weren't constantly being specially bred and hybridized to make them sweeter and sweeter.)

We unfortunately veered away from having a pretty good understanding of what made us fat. One of the great mistakes made was concluding that glucose (a simple sugar) is the best of all fuels. That conclusion was reached when we learned the body chooses to prioritize it, to metabolize it *before* other possible fuels such as fats or proteins. But what Mr. Taubes and Drs. Lustig, Bernstein and Perlmutter all say is that the body prioritizes sugars, metabolizes them first – not because it's a better fuel – but because it wants to lower the amount present in the blood.

Now, how harmful it is to a particular individual depends on some variables: how much sugar you actually consume is in that food, how much fiber is along with it in that food, how much sugar you've eaten over your lifetime and how your own, unique genetic makeup has set you up to handle it. In this context again, I'm no longer referring to table sugar, but to all carbohydrates, because, iterating, once in the bloodstream as sugar, your body will immediately try to rid itself of it. How?

By using insulin. Insulin is a hormone, the body's regulator of blood sugar. When sugar first arrives in the mouth, the tongue tells the brain "sweet" and signals the pancreas to start producing insulin (in fact, if you *think* about the coconut cream pie you're about to eat, the pancreas gears up in advance). *Hey, pancreas! Looks like some sugar's on the way; get ready!* So the pancreas starts insulin coursing through the bloodstream, telling every cell to open up, take in the sugar, and metabolize it with priority. *And . . .* (this is the really nasty part) at the same time, insulin *immediately* takes roughly 20 – 25% of those sugar calories and converts them to fat cells. This is critical to understand, so let me state it again, as described by Dr. Lustig:

If you – average person – need 2000 calories to get through your day's activities, and on this day you consume 2000 calories from "complex carbohydrates," as many as 500 of those calories will not be burned; they'll be turned into fat *before* you can burn them, *even though you balanced calories consumed with calories your activities required!* We all have some fat cells, they're important, and they represent a good source of fuel. But so long as you're consuming carbs – sugars – the fats won't be metabolized until the level of blood sugar is reduced to a safe level, and any additional carbs you consume will be subject to the very same formulaic conversion. If you're an obese person, you've got loads of available fuel (fat cells), but you can't get at it; it's locked away, and so long as you're consuming more carbs, more of them *continue* to get locked away as fat.

Sounds like a pretty bad trap to be in, and it is. *But wait – there's more!* The reason is, over time, we become increasingly insulin *resistant*, that is to say, over time we require *more* insulin to handle the *same* amount of carbs. So over time, as we become more and more resistant to insulin, we have to release more of it to handle the same amount of sugars, and the more insulin that's released, the higher the percentage of those carbs will be converted to fat!

Oh, yeah, here's another little nasty fact: since you – the average person who needs 2000 calories that day – *didn't actually get to burn* those 2000 calories, but instead parked some away as fat, you're going to still be hungry because you didn't get to use your needed 2000 calories. Your hunger is not a weakness on your part, it's simply a biological imperative. You'll probably feel run down, since you're short on fuel, but you will be hungry.

What about will power? Sure, will-power can overcome hunger pangs for a day, maybe two, maybe a week, a month or two, or even longer than that. But a consistent deficit in calories is, by definition, starvation, and all human beings, as creatures of biology, cannot starve indefinitely . . . we're hard-wired to eat when hungry.

What's the lesson to take from this? Counting calories doesn't work; countless studies have shown this, though sadly, it's still often quoted as fact. But, reducing your intake of carbohydrates (sugars) will reduce insulin production and turn down or even turn off the automatic fat-storage machine. Without the carbs, or with carbs that arrive with lots of fiber, you can eat until you're satisfied, not leave the table hungry, and your body can burn the fat that's always circulating in our blood, always available.

Wait a minute, wait a minute...didn't you earlier write how when trying to stop eating carbs you succeeded once but then failed twice, because you craved them so?

I did, indeed. As I wrote, that's exactly why, when I first learned of Taubes' book and gave it a cursory look-see to learn what it said, I was skeptical. Here's the difference between then and now: During my preceding attempts, I tried to *remove* carbs from my diet. When I assembled and gleaned an understanding of all this new information, I ate carbs . . . I *still* eat carbs; what changed was the form they're in. Hey, I like a plate of spaghetti as much as anyone, and never again having pasta didn't strike me as a recipe for success. I had only to make a very simple change: when I eat spaghetti now, it's *whole-grain spaghetti*.

Remember fiber? It's what they scrub out of most spaghetti and macaroni, and also out of that nice, white rice and that nice, white sandwich bread. I still eat rice, too, it's just not the processed stuff.

Oh, more on that topic, those two failed attempts at carbs reduction . . . I wrote that on the second and third attempts, my insides were *screaming,* that I felt as though I were Frank Sinatra's heroin-addicted character in "The Man With the Golden Arm." It turns out that isn't just a useful metaphor, but instead has real truth. Gluten is the sticky stuff that holds bread together, it's what makes pizza so good. Gluten-free has become topical; it's said that approximately 30% of us have "Celiac Disease," a condition where gluten cannot be tolerated at all, and that's resulted in an increasing number of foods boasting themselves to be "Gluten-Free."

So? If I'm not among the 30%, what's the big deal?

Well, here's interesting news: When gluten is digested, Gluteomorphin is formed. Gluteomorphin – also known as Gliadorphin – is an opiod (think morphine) bound with gluten. It stimulates the same areas of the brain as do other opioids, sometimes creating an addiction as real as any other. Turns out my insides *were* screaming!

Here's another thing to keep in mind as you consider what to eat. In department stores, at consumer shows, on infomercials and shopping channels, you can find very fancy juicers for sale. Juicing is *terrific*; extracting the fiber from fresh vegetable will let you drink in more nutrients and vitamins and enzymes than you possibly could if you tried to eat so many of those veggies in one sitting. Could you eat three or four large plates filled with spinach and kale and broccoli and cabbage and Brussels sprouts in one sitting? That's a lot, so probably not. But if you juiced them, you could drink all their juice. However, it's wiser to *not* juice fruits, except perhaps in small quantities, maybe mixed in with the vegetables. Removing the fiber leaves just the sugary water (remember the OJ); you *need* the fiber from fruits. There are blenders powerful enough to pulverize veggies and fruits; since they don't remove the fiber, you're probably ok.

Look, I'm not an absolute zealot about this. I won't drink apple juice (no fiber), but I'll eat an apple, which I wouldn't have during my Atkins attempts. I have completely sworn off potato chips and cakes, but once in a great while – a special occasion, say, Thanksgiving, I'll eat a helping of mashed potatoes and pumpkin pie and now and again I'll make vichyssoise.

And especially in the heat of summer, I drink beer. But for the most part, the carbs that I consume are in their whole form, i.e., they have fiber (yes, I know, no fiber in beer, alas). If you eat as I now do, my guess is you'll lose weight. But remember, I may have had Archie Bunker's shape, but I was never close to being morbidly obese. If your weight issues are more severe, or if you're more insulin-resistant, you may need to be more strict in limiting your intake of carbs-without-fiber than I; maybe much more severe, or maybe you can just leave out the beer. But once you do change *how* you get your calories rather than *count* them, you'll be amazed how quickly you'll shed pounds. Best of all, you won't feel as though you're being punished.

One final word about sugars, and I'll be very brief. I'd mentioned previously that Dr. Lustig particularly vilifies high-fructose corn syrup, and in his more recent lecture, "Fat Chance: Fructose 2.0," he does so even more sharply. Here's why: Glucose, the energy molecule in table sugar, is a fuel, and can be metabolized by every cell in the body. Fructose is the "sweet" molecule in table sugar, and it can only be metabolized in the liver. Moreover, it doesn't drive satiety, the feeling of "having had enough." When you feel you've eaten enough, the hormone leptin is produced and is seen by the brain as the signal to stop eating. But high fructose corn syrup *doesn't* cause leptin to be produced, so the brain still thinks it needs more fuel, re-introducing the biological imperative to eat. Dr. Lustig sees HFCS's introduction in the mid-seventies as one of the most important drivers of our collective rush to obesity, as he explains in both of those youtube lectures.

MYTH NUMBER TWO: EXERCISE MORE AND EAT LESS . . . THAT'S HOW TO LOSE WEIGHT.

This goes hand-in-glove with counting calories. If my intake remains the same, but I burn more, how could I not lose weight? There is an element of truth to this, but the difference it makes to weight loss negligible. As we've seen, it's not the number of calories taken in, it's their form. Fewer carbs, or slower carb-absorption because of fiber means lower blood sugar; less blood sugar means less insulin; less insulin means you can burn fat as fuel. But if we lower our intake of carbs, wouldn't exercise then accelerate our weight loss? Perhaps a bit, but not significantly, for two main reasons. One, exercising will probably make you hungrier than you would have been had you not exercised, so you'll eat more. The phrase "work up an appetite" isn't a cliché for nothing.

But much more important: To have much impact on how much you weigh, you'd have to exercise far more than you likely suspect. It is true, exercise will burn calories and build muscles. It's also true that, even at rest, muscle tissue metabolizes calories faster than fat tissue. Most important: exercise is good for you; it's one of the best – maybe *the* best – things you can do to improve your health! It will benefit your cardio-vascular system (stronger heart, lower blood pressure) your pulmonary system (lungs) it'll improve your mood, likely your brain cognition and even your sex-life. (Hmmm...so maybe I *will* do more than get up and change the channel!) So by all means, do! Exercise! Yes yes yes! It will help you become healthier and fitter. Uhm . . . just don't expect your exercise to help you lose very *much* weight.

Here's why, here's what they never tell you: According to *www.medicinenet.com* a 150 pound man burns 100 calories walking a mile at an average walking speed; other sources vary, but not by much. If the person weighs more or less, then more or fewer calories would be burned for the same distance. When dieticians tell you to exercise more and eat less to lose weight, they never seem to get around to telling you *how much* exercise you need. Do you know how many calories equal a pound? Have you ever read it, or heard it discussed when exercise is talked about in relation to weight loss? Maybe . . . but probably not, because the answer would quite undercut the persuasive value of the exercise regimen – or equipment they're selling – as a means to lose weight. Since I've learned this, I've asked many individuals this question, and have never found anyone who's known.

The answer is, one pound is equal to 3,500 calories. This means, if our 150 pound man wants to lose *just one pound* through exercise, he'd have to walk a mile each day for 35 days . . . over a month! Or 2 miles for 17 days and 1 mile on the 18th day . . . or in whatever permutations applied to the goal he selected. And *that* assumes he doesn't eat any more than he did before beginning his walking regimen . . . you know, that "working up an appetite" thing. If I'd set about to lose my 40+ pounds of excess weight by walking a mile a day, it would have taken me over 46 months . . . nearly 4 years.[2] These first two myths are joined at the hip,

---

[2] In truth, it likely would have taken *over* 4 years, because while I would have begun the regimen weighing in at over 150 lbs., as my weight fell (albeit slowly), it would have meant that I'd no longer be burning *quite* 100 calories per mile.

and as I said, it's awfully hard to resist what seems so obviously true. One might suppose, or at least hope, that those who are in the fields of medicine and nutrition would be less swayed by that which seems *intuitively* true than by what the evidence actually *shows*. But when you've been taught something for years and years, have believed it for years and years and perhaps even passed it on to others for years and years – especially if you've been viewed as an authority – it's only human nature to be reluctant to backpedal and say, "Uhm . . . sorry about that."

Gary Taubes points this out again and again in his book "Why We Get Fat." He analyzes studies made over decades, dissects them and finds errors; sometimes the errors are in the study's protocol, sometimes in their conclusions. The first time I read his book I was stunned by one sentence in particular, and sadly, it perfectly illustrates how incorrect beliefs, even without supporting evidence, are so resolutely clung to.

In his third chapter, "The Elusive Benefits of Exercise," he brings our attention to "guidelines to physical activity and health" published jointly in August, 2007, by The American Heart Association and the American College of Sports Medicine. In it, the authors recommended thirty minutes of moderately vigorous physical activity five days a week, as necessary to "maintain and promote health." But the sentence I found so stunning was a paragraph later, when Taubes quotes the authors:

> "It is reasonable to assume that persons with relatively *high* daily energy expenditures would be *less likely to gain weight* over time, compared with those who have low energy expenditures. **So far, data to support this hypothesis are not particularly compelling."** [Emphasis mine.]

I say again, exercise! It's good for you, it *is* important for your overall health; just don't expect it to contribute much to your weight loss.

MYTH NUMBER THREE: FAT IS BAD FOR YOU, IT'S THE ULTIMATE ENEMY

Drs. Lustig and Perlmutter, as well as Mr. Taubes, all take aim at this myth, but when they do, they're not saying, "Hey, go ahead and eat lots of fat, it's all harmless." The reason they don't is there are many kinds of fats, some good, some bad, and the differences between them are complex. I've read, listened, asked my friend Dr. Mike to help me better understand, and despite that, I still don't personally have a deep enough grasp to explain the differences to you in a way that would satisfy a science major. I could quote terms or expressions or sentences – fatty acids, long-chain fatty acids, itty-bitty chains, saturated fats, unsaturated fats, trans fats, single bond, double bond, auto bondo, whatever . . . and then I could quote the definitions. But you know what? No matter how well I might learn to parrot these terms, I don't really understand the chemistry; I'm a performer, a musician. But you know what else? It's ok, *I don't have to understand them;* I only have to know enough to choose the good ones and avoid the bad.

If that's true, how did we come to believe this "All fat is bad" paradigm?

That's a fair question, especially when we review what we *used to* know versus what we "know" *now*. Until recently, but for a long time before that, it was the absolutely accepted medical dogma that starchy and sweet foods were what made you fat. As Taubes points out, the famous baby doctor, Dr. Benjamin Spock, wrote in 1946: "The amount of plain, starchy foods (cereals, breads, potatoes) taken is what determines, in the case of most people, how much [weight] they gain or lose."

In his book, Taubes also cites how through the 19th century, everyone knew that starches were what made you fat, and that knowledge remained in place through most of the 20th century. He tells us how, in the 1950's, an obese person admitted to the hospital was immediately put on a diet that restricted starches, sweets and all things made from flour . . . that, according to documents he examined from the medical schools at Harvard, Cornell and Stanford.

Both he and Dr. Lustig then relate how Ancel Keys, a Minnesota epidemiologist, in 1980 published the "Seven Countries Study." In the study, and based on evidence that both Taubes and Lustig consider flawed, Keys connected dietary fat to cardiovascular disease. Meanwhile, through the 1970's, it was learned that dietary fat raised a person's LDL, or "bad cholesterol." We'll discuss cholesterol more in the next section, but because of these perceptions, fat was quickly demonized. Foods suddenly became available in "low fat" or "no fat" varieties; butter was thought bad, margarine good, and whole milk was thought less healthy than 2%, though 1% was better, and skim milk was obviously best of all.

This shift created a problem for the giant food corporations. Look, I wouldn't say Food Inc. is out to get you; I *would* say it's out to get your dollars. Food companies are in business, and if you're going to buy a food, whether it's ice cream, cookies, frozen vegetables, cereal, pickles, cheese or hot dogs, there are hundreds of choices available and the food companies want you to choose theirs.

Now, you've probably said, or heard someone say, "How come everything I *like* to eat is bad for me?" That so often seems true because it's fat that gives food flavor and texture; without fat, foods are often about as appetizing as old shingles, and food that tastes like old shingles just isn't going to sell very well. The food companies had to find ways to be able to say "low-fat" or "fat-free" *and still make the foods taste good!* The obvious way was to add sugars, in whatever form. Corn syrup, molasses, maltose, dextrose . . . these are all sugars you can find on the labels of so many foods (sometimes they just call it sugar . . . what a concept!). Over the last decades, though, high fructose corn syrup has become the sweetener of choice, largely because it's cheap. If you recall our previous discussion of sugar and how it leads to insulin resistance and automatic fat storage, it's not hard to see how we got our initial shove into the obesity epidemic.

Ok, the sugar's bad, I can see that. Even so, we should still avoid the fat, right?

No and yes. Yes and no. It depends. Honest, I'm not vacillating. It depends on what kind of fat we're talking about, and there are several kinds. In general:

SATURATED FATS are derived mostly from animal products and are solid at room temperature. The marbling in your steak is a saturated fat. There are also a few plants from which saturated fats can be derived, such as coconut oil and palm oil.

UNSATURATED FATS are liquid at room temperature, and there are two kinds, mono-unsaturated and poly-unsaturated. Of the two types, mono is probably better for you. Olive oil is a mono-unsaturated fat, as are the fats in peanut oil, canola oil and avocados. Examples of poly-unsaturated fats include the oils made from corn, cottonseed, soybean, safflower and sesame.

TRANS FATS are, in the words of Dr. Lustig, "the devil incarnate and will kill you." Well, he made that clear enough, there's no mistaking what he thinks of them, but what are they and where are they found? They're also known as partially-hydrogenated vegetable oils, and that's exactly what they are: vegetable oil treated with hydrogen gas, which then makes it more solid, but still allows it to melt easily. Trans fats were invented in the early 20th century and led to the development of vegetable shortening, margarine and other products. Not only is it cheap, but it adds stability (pronounced "shelf life") to foods. Shelf life, of course, means that foods can ride in trucks and sit on grocery shelves far longer without going bad. And of course that means, if it doesn't sell quickly it doesn't have to be thrown away in the garbage; throwing your product away in the garbage is a thoroughly efficient method of reducing profit.

OMEGA-3 FATTY ACIDS are essential to our good health, critical to brain function, and sadly, cannot be manufactured by our bodies; we have to eat them. Good sources for Omega-3's include cold water fish like salmon; they're also in flax seed, soy and walnuts.

Those are basic definitions of fats. More complex explanations are readily available for those who want to understand the complex chemical bonds involved, but these basic definitions were sufficient for me to know which to eat and which to avoid. But back to the myth, and the question of whether fats are good or bad.

I'd answered that previously with "yes and no," and the definitions themselves offer some insight why I did. Omega-3's are necessary; trans fats are off the table. But there's more to it.

We *need* to have some fat in our bodies, and not just the Omega-3's. Fat cushions organs and keeps fat-soluble Vitamins like A, D, E and K in the body. It also helps keep our skin healthy and aids in metabolism.

And it is also a very good fuel! Fat is constantly being released into our blood from its storage in our fat cells, where, riding along in the bloodstream, it's always there, constantly available for our cells to burn. Of course, as we've seen, if we introduce sugar into our blood, the body will more quickly burn the sugar and ignore the fat, but the body's priority to reduce blood sugar does not diminish fat's own quality as a fuel. It's a very efficient way of getting fuel, too. One gram of fat has nine calories, versus four calories for both proteins and carbs.

All of the sources I've repeatedly cited – Drs. Perlmutter, Bernstein and Lustig plus science writer Gary Taubes – agree that our modern American diet is upside down. They unanimously point to the fact that human beings evolved as hunter-gatherers, eating meats, as well as berries, roots and other vegetation as they could find. They also agree that the relatively recent advent of agriculture – only the last ten thousand years or so – is a mere blip in our evolutionary timeline, arguing that we *didn't* evolve to eat cereals and grains. Moreover, they point to the last fifty years or so, when carbohydrates (cereals and grains), and particularly *processed carbs* became an ever-increasing part of our diets while we shied away from fats; they offer that shift as the prime cause of our obesity epidemic and its associated ills such as heart disease and diabetes.

So, which foods are ok to eat? The answer is relatively simple, and as my personal story illustrates, doesn't require a complete grasp of bio-chemistry and how fatty acids chain together. I can't diagram a chemical bond, but I can choose fats that occur naturally. I eat and enjoy steaks and pork chops. I eat chicken, and *don't* remove the skin. (*Fat is a good fuel!*) I drink whole milk and use cream in my coffee, but avoid artificial creamers. (We do need *some* sugar; milk contains lactose, a sugar, and I eat carbs that come with fiber.) I cook with butter, olive oil and coconut oil, and will deep-fry chicken wings in peanut oil. I never use margarine. It's pretty simple, really, and best of all, I eat all I want; I don't leave the table hungry . . . I'm not a glutton, but I eat until I'm full.

Finally, for a slightly different reason, I want to return to trans fats, the hydrogenated oils that could once be found in almost any commercially baked product, and which for years was used for frying. There's no disagreement that they're bad, and for years, pressure's been mounting for them to be removed from the marketplace. In 2006 the Food and Drug Administration required trans fats be included on nutrition labels, in 2007 New York City banned them from restaurants, and in November, 2013, the FDA announced it would move to ban them altogether, beginning with a two month period of collecting data, while inviting comment. As I write this, that period of data collection has closed.

The data collection is being followed by a period of evaluation, and if that results in a final decision to ban trans fats, a deadline will be issued for completely phasing them out. It won't be immediate, because manufacturers will be allowed some time to reformulate their products.

All of that is welcome, but it's not all you need to know. As we've seen, trans fats have come under fire for over a decade, and if you walk your grocery's aisles, you'll easily find products that boast, "0 trans fats!" On other products, the packaging may not *boast* it has no trans fats, but if you randomly choose to read the labels on things like hamburger buns or cookies or pretzels you'll routinely see the nutrition breakdown telling you:

Total Grams of Fat: X

Grams of Saturated Fat: X

Grams of Trans Fat: **0**

Grams of Polyunsaturated Fat: X

Grams of Monounsaturated Fat: X

You'll also see how many grams of sugars, fibers, proteins, cholesterol and calories the product contains. If you do this, you'll be *extremely* hard pressed to find *any* of them with even *one* gram of trans fats (which is why in the example I specified 0 for trans fats). Great news, then, no?

Well . . . ~*sigh*~ . . . here's another dirty little secret, and this one is *really* dirty: When it says "0 Trans Fats" the product might *still contain trans fats.* Legally.

How can that be?

That's a really good question, isn't it? See, when in 2006 the FDA ordered nutrition labels include the amount of trans fats, it became necessary to define 0 grams of trans fats.

Huh? Hello...0 means zero, naught, nada; what do you mean? What else **could** *it mean?*

In an age when "zero-tolerance" is a term generally understood, it is nevertheless *not* the term that describes "0 Trans Fats." Whether it was heavy lobbying, generous contributions, lavish parties, naiveté or just a pitch delivered by an incredibly persuasive salesman, the FDA agreed to allow the term "0 Trans Fats" to be used in the labeling if . . . wait for it . . . *the amount of trans fats was a half gram or less . . . <u>per serving</u>!*

Per serving! PER SERVING!! **PER SERVING!!!!** Do you see what this allows? All of the numbers you read when you pick up that bag of donuts or cookies, the grams of fats, sugars, fiber and the calories, too –

all of them – only apply to the amount "per serving" . . . you know, the amount you'd eat at "one sitting."

And now you know why – on so many products, whether canned peaches or baked beans or cookies – the serving size on the label is appropriate for a four-year-old. I looked at a package of commonly-found sandwich cookies. It listed no trans fat per serving, but the serving size was two cookies . . . *two*! Wait a minute, you know what? I take it back; that's not even enough for a four-year-old! A package of frozen pinto beans listed a serving size as a half-cup;   frozen broccoli listed its serving size as one full cup (ah, but frozen broccoli doesn't have stuff that needs to be hidden, does it?); canned corn a half cup; a can of soup (add milk or water) listed a serving size as a half cup.

If you don't already know how little that is, find a measuring cup and fill it to the half line;   *that's a serving of soup?* I put water into a modest bowl, and filled it to what I thought represented a typical bowl of soup. I then measured it; it came out to a little over a cup and a half, more than three times the "serving size" suggested by the label.

You see what they're doing, don't you? "Serving size" is completely arbitrary, there are no rules, it's set by the food manufacturers, and food manufacturers aren't worried about you planning how much to buy for your dinner party. *"Hmmm . . . six guests, plus me and my date, that's eight . . . ok, I see servings per container is four, so I guess I need two cans"* (or packages, or bags, or whatever). They're not calculating "serving size" based on how many actual servings it is in real life, they're calculating "serving size" by determining how big it can be before it trips over the limit, i.e., before the trans fats would exceed half a gram! If the FDA does move forward with a total ban on trans fats, I don't know if that loophole will remain. One would hope not, but it will bear watching.

MYTH NUMBER FOUR: CHOLES-TEROL IS BAD AND CAUSES HEART DISEASE

This just about as firmly entrenched as is the myth about counting calories, its origins coincide with our belief that fat is bad, and sadly, although studies have *not* found any correlation between high cholesterol levels and mortality, it lives on. The myth has made billions of dollars for pharmaceutical companies because they sell statin drugs, the drugs that lower cholesterol. Look, "Big Pharma" didn't create the myth, but if there is a widely-held belief that lowering cholesterol is a good thing, their labs will be happy to find ways to help you do it with pills. But is lowering cholesterol even a good thing at all?

First of all, no study has ever found cholesterol causes heart disease. Instead, the original conclusion that it did was formed along these lines:

1) Overweight men are more likely to die of heart disease than those who are not; true.

2) Cholesterol levels are higher in overweight men than in those who are not; true.

3) Conclusion: Higher cholesterol levels must cause heart disease.

Clear enough.

Except it's not clear at all. Drawing that conclusion is no more logical than saying,

1) Sometimes it rains hard; true.

2) When it rains hard, robins are in my yard;
except in winter, true.

3) Conclusion: Hard rain must cause robins.

In both examples, of course, the first and second
statements are true, but the conclusions merely take
notice of co-incidence, not cause. Some facts:

- Cholesterol is vital to all mammalian life, an
essential structural component of their cell
membranes.

- Cholesterol is necessary for all our cells, but
it's especially essential for brain health. In
adults, the brain is roughly 2 - 3% of our
body weight, but it contains *25% of the
body's cholesterol.*

- While there is no study showing elevated
cholesterol levels cause heart disease, there
are several studies that show diet doesn't
affect cholesterol levels anyway! You're
likely familiar with the term "risk factor."
That term came from the *Framingham
Heart Study,* which began in 1948 in
Framingham, MA. It continues still, now

on its third generation of participants. It has consistently shown that blood cholesterol levels for those who ate above-average amounts of cholesterol were virtually identical to those who ate below-average amounts of cholesterol. That's because if we reduce the amount of cholesterol we eat, our bodies will simply make more.

Cholesterol also developed a bad rap because of studies done on rabbits and chickens. They were force-fed high levels of cholesterol, and yes, it was positively proven that they developed arteriosclerosis. But to extrapolate from that study done on rabbits and chickens a conclusion that cholesterol is bad for humans is simply bad science, *very* bad science. *All* it proves is that rabbits and chickens on a high-cholesterol diet develop arteriosclerosis, nothing more. But rabbits and chickens didn't evolve as meat eaters (chickens do eat insects, but there isn't much cholesterol in them), so the comparison is invalid.

In 2012, a book called "The Great Cholesterol Myth" was published. It was co-authored by Dr. Stephen Sinatra, (M.D.) a cardiologist, and Dr. Jonny Bowden (Ph.D.) a nutritionist. In their book they strongly argue that the case against cholesterol is weak. When they appeared on "The Dr. Oz Show" in December of 2012, Dr. Oz, himself a cardiologist, said at the show's onset, "Today is a game changer, it's the most important show I've ever done on cholesterol."

It's another book I'd suggest you read; you can also watch their appearance on the Oz show on-line. But in short, what they said was that cholesterol numbers don't matter, that inflammation of the blood vessels is what matters. And what causes inflammation of the blood vessels? According to Dr. Sinatra, it's sugar. (Hmmm . . . methinks a clear pattern has emerged . . . *ain't nobody sayin' nothin' nice about sugar.*)

It's interesting to note, too, that neurologist Dr. David Perlmutter, whom I've already cited in this book, also appeared on Dr. Oz about a year later. Dr. Perlmutter showed Dr. Oz what he considered bad foods; they included potatoes, corn, and even whole wheat bread. He doesn't believe there are any good carbs, period. He doesn't say avoid them at all cost, but does say they should be *very* limited. He then showed Dr. Oz his choices for healthy foods, which many good fats (when he said butter was good, the audience spontaneously burst into applause!). A year previously, when Drs. Sinatra and Bowden were on his show, Dr. Oz was open minded, but clearly had reservations; after all, he'd spent his entire professional life warning of cholesterol's dangers. This time, as the discussion between the two ended, Dr. Oz told Dr. Perlmutter, on camera, that "Heart doctors like myself are starting to buy into this idea." You also can find Dr. Perlmutter's Dr. Oz appearance on-line.

Some final words on cholesterol . . . we hear of "good" cholesterol (High-density lipoprotein, or HDL) and "bad" cholesterol (Low-density lipoprotein, or LDL). But it turns out even that distinction isn't so clear, because there's more than one type of LDL. One type is large and buoyant, the other is small and non-buoyant. Turns out, even those who subscribe to the idea that LDL is bad agree that the large and buoyant kind is actually *not* bad.

MYTH NUMBER FIVE: A HEALTHY DIET IS REPRESENTED BY THE USDA'S FOOD PYRAMID

Actually, the food pyramid died, replaced by a plate. If you Google MyPyramid or MyPlate, you'll find that MyPlate replaced MyPyramid in 2011, and was based on the newer USDA guidelines issued in 2010. But it doesn't matter which one you look at, the information remains flawed. The base of the pyramid is made of grains: bread, rice, pasta, cereals. Obviously all the sources I cite in this book would vehemently disagree with that. In the MyPlate image, vegetables represent the largest portion of the plate (but it makes no distinction between starchy and non-starchy veggies), with grains almost as large. In either, fruits get a significant share, with smaller portions of dairy and meats recommended. And at the top of the pyramid, the stuff you should eat the least of, according to the thinking of the time, were fats, oils and sweets. Is your head spinning yet? During his appearance on "The Peoples Pharmacy," Dr. Perlmutter said, "I'm not turning the food pyramid upside down, it *is* upside down. I'm trying to put it back to where it belongs."

Look, if, as you should, you watch/listen/read the various authors and authorities I've mentioned through this book, you'll discover they're not in absolute and complete lockstep. That's not surprising; the evidence is being viewed through different prisms. Dr. Lustig says fruit with fiber is ok, and also allows whole grain bread. But as an endocrinologist, he's viewing these data from the perspective of how weight is regulated by hormones, and he especially hates high fructose corn syrup. Neurologist Dr. Perlmutter says that all the carbs are bad, but his perspective is from one who views carbs' effects on the brain. Gary Taubes says that pineapple or watermelon (*very* sweet, with little fiber) would likely cause more problems than a pear. Dr. Bernstein's point of view, since he treats diabetes, isn't from carbs' effects on the brain, but instead its effects on blood glucose levels and how it relates to those with diabetes, which is often caused by obesity.

But all of them uniformly declare that carbs – remember, they're all ultimately sugar – wreak havoc on our health, and are largest cause of the enormous increases we've seen in chronic diseases. And it's certainly true that obesity itself is the prime driver for so many other chronic conditions. I'd agree – and my own experience has proven to my own satisfaction – that whether it's MyPyramid or MyPlate, the conventional wisdom isn't wise at all.

If you're interested in exploring the forces that gave rise to the food pyramid and its incarnations, you could read Denise Minger's "Death by Food Pyramid: How Shoddy Science, Sketchy Politics and Shady Special Interests Have Ruined Our Health."

5. IT'S A WRAP!

So, is this "the Atkins Diet" again? And you often mentioned "our ancestors," and how we evolved . . . is it "Paleo?"

No, not quite, although there are obvious similarities.

Well, shouldn't I be worried? Back in its heyday, weren't they calling the "Atkins Diet" a "<u>killer</u> <u>diet</u>?"

I believe that until the current conventional wisdom dies its inevitable death, there will be an ever-decreasing number of individuals who will defend that conventional wisdom, and right now they're still in the majority. Remember, there is a lot of money at stake, and money always influences. I'm not declaring the whole system is corrupt, merely that perspective always mandates subjectivity, even if unintentional. If exercise is promoted *exclusively* for its well-warranted health benefits, but *not* for weight-loss, doesn't that winnow from the number of prospective customers for exercise equipment those who would buy it to just lose weight? I mean, yes, some people, like my brother, exercise because they know it helps keep them healthy, they like the way it makes them feel and they'll always choose to do so. But, other individuals exercise only because they've been told it's how to get slim. If that latter group learned that exercising won't do much for their weight-loss, they would no longer be very good prospects for home gyms and the like, would they? Which could mean that gyms and exercise equipment manufacturers might not be enthusiastic disseminators of this information.

Still, do your own homework. Ask your physician, and to reiterate, if he or she holds onto the old paradigm, show him or her these data. If you or your physician is concerned about the effects of fats on your heart, let me one more time return to Gary Taubes, author of "Why We Get Fat." During his August, 2011 appearance on "The Peoples Pharmacy," and in his book, he cites studies in which individuals were randomly assigned to one of two groups: one group would eat "heart healthy" diets: salads, fruits, vegetables and cereals, while avoiding much meat or fat, as recommended by the American Heart Association. The other group would eat an Atkins-like diet, where meats and fatty foods could be eaten freely, but carbohydrates were limited. According to Taubes, in each study, the Atkins groups lost more weight. If you've read this far, that shouldn't surprise, but if your physician questions the wisdom of eating these fatty foods *despite* the impressive record of weight loss, this should be eye-opening, even eye-popping: the Atkins-like groups also ended up with the *healthier cardio-profiles*, i.e., their risk factors for heart disease were *lower* than the AHA's "heart healthy diet" group!

Or how about this: Dr. Perlmutter, during his appearance on "The Peoples Pharmacy," spoke of a 2013 report in "The New England Journal of Medicine." He described an interventional trial of three groups: one ate the typical American diet high in carbs; the second ate the Mediterranean Diet; the third ate a modified Mediterranean Diet, the modification being increased fats. The trial was discontinued in just a little over four and a half years because the third group, the one eating more fats showed a *30% risk reduction of developing either stroke, heart attack or death!* The researchers saw such a stark difference they thought it was unfair to the first two groups to let the trial go on.

If you choose to – and you should – listen to the podcasts you'll learn more and in greater detail than I present here. If you also watch the videos you'll learn still more. And if you take the time to read the books I mention and others as well, you'll come away with as much – probably more – knowledge about all this than I have. When your friends start asking you how *you* did it, you'll be able to explain as I've tried to here. But what I've written here, while true, is merely the tip of the iceberg; as you listen, read and view, you'll be fascinated by some of the things you'll discover. An example: in his "Fructose 2.0" lecture, Dr. Lustig quotes a study by the American Diabetes Association from March, 2013. The study revealed that diabetes alone cost the US $245 billion in 2012 alone. And obesity is one of the prime drivers toward diabetes and hypertension, too. In Gary Taubes' book, you'll learn how genetics can be the determinate for *where* on your body your extra fat gets stored. Again, if you do the research, you'll be amazed by the things you'll find. But for now, here is my summary, including a few extra health tidbits.

- Counting calories doesn't work.

- Limit carbs, yes, but you needn't eliminate them. When they *are* consumed, make sure they've got lots of fiber by eating the whole fruit, bread or pasta made from whole wheat, and unprocessed rice. Fiber delays the carbs' absorption into the blood, reducing the spike in your blood glucose level, which then reduces your insulin response. Remember, *avoiding* carbs is what caused my feeling like the "Man With the Golden Arm." I *do* consume carbs, just not many, and they nearly always have fiber.

- Fat is a good fuel, assuming you eat the good ones, the *real* ones as are found in nature.

- Meat is good, and I eat a good deal of it. Fish is probably better because it's richer in omega-3 fats. If you do eat beef, grass fed is better than grain fed. Cattle didn't evolve to eat grain, and while it may fatten them up (hmm, carbs make them fat, too?), it's also likely to cause GI tract sores, sores that might become infected were it not for the all-but-universal administration of antibiotics (a good reason to choose grass fed and organic). Back to fish: fish is good, especially cold-water fish, and the best of those are probably fresh-caught.

- If you do have something sweet, but can choose between something with sugar or something with high-fructose corn syrup, choose the sugar. I mentioned earlier that Dr. Lustig points out that fructose can only be metabolized by the liver. He's seen cases of teenage boys who needed *liver transplants* because of all the sodas they drank, sodas sweetened with HFCS (it's metabolized in the liver the same way it metabolized alcohol, thus leading to fatty liver disease). Recall, too that another reason he detests it is that it doesn't cause a sense of satiety, of "being full." At least sugar does that.

- Consider this, too: *"Avoid sugar, huh? Ok . . . I can drink artificially sweetened drinks then?"* Not so much. Personally, I hate the taste of artificial sweeteners, and I also don't trust stuff that's manufactured in a lab. But beyond that, remember that a sweet *taste e*vokes an insulin response. But if your blood sugar is already at a safe level when you then evoke an insulin response, the insulin will indeed do its thing, it will lower your blood sugar. But if it didn't need to be lowered . . . the result will be blood sugar that's too *low*. By definition, that's hypoglycemia, and at the very least you'll feel sleepy and/or hungry.

The advantages of eating as I do are: I lost the weight and I never feel hungry. I can eat as much (non-starchy) vegetables, meat and eggs as I want and not gain weight. Eating this way, I get that leptin signal of satiety, the sense that, "Ok, I'm not hungry anymore." If I become hungry mid-afternoon, I don't need to summon will power, but instead eat! Maybe a couple of slices of cheese (real cheese, not some processed, who-knows-what's-in-it "cheese-food") or nuts, or pepperoni slices, maybe an apple.

Remember, it's carbs that get insulin flowing, and insulin automatically turns some of the carbs into fat. If you – like I was – are overweight but not obese, you may be able to enjoy – as I do – the occasional food that has carbs even without fiber. I do drink beer. Alas, no fiber, though it's rich in carbs; but it's an exception and inasmuch as my weight has stabilized where I want it, for me it works. I also drink some milk (whole milk), and it obviously lacks fiber, too, but does have the sugar lactose; my metabolism allows that, while yours may not. Again, if you are obese, or if you have a genetic, family history toward obesity, as

Gary Taubes in his book explains *does happen*, you may have to minimize carbs more strictly than I.

I don't sweeten my coffee any more, and as I'd said, it's the single element I miss most since changing what I eat, but I'm pleased that I can allow that beer and wine. The bottom line is, watch your results, and adjust accordingly.

In that vein, whole fruits are generally ok for me; they may or may not be ok for you (though, again, there's obviously not much fiber in watermelon). Certainly, by now you understand that fruit juices are out of the question, but even whole fruits give me at least *some* pause, based on Dr. Perlmutter's assertions that carbs can lead to a shrinking brain, Alzheimer's and dementia. I know I can't as readily recall a fact or a name as quickly I once did (I was absolutely *great* playing the home versions of *Jeopardy!* . . . must have been all those arcane things I read). If I can get some of that back, I'm willing to reduce my intake of carbs a bit more. But again, I'm not a fanatic. And I also keep in mind Dr. Lustig's words, that sweets were supposed to be a treat, maybe once a week, not every meal. I've also written that I'll once in a while enjoy mashed potatoes, or a holiday dessert. I may also have vichyssoise, which has potatoes, but which I love and consider to be a delicacy. So I have it once in a while;

vichyssoise gets to be on my table maybe twice a year, as a treat.

I used to be the "Will Rogers of pizza;" I never met one I didn't like. And it's true, pizza might have landed *ahead* of sweetened coffee on the list of things I no longer eat/drink, but miss. It might have, except, unlike sweetened coffee, I do once in a while have a pizza, *but:* it's pizza whose crust is made from whole grain flour. I can then load it up with the cheeses and meats and sauces I enjoy. Is it quite as yummy? In all honesty, no, but it is close, and I'm having pizza! I don't feel deprived, and . . . I'm svelte!

Vegetables are excellent, they take up room, helping you feel full, they provide vitamins and enzymes and can be the best source of fiber. But I avoid corn because it's full of starch (we call it "sweet corn," after all) as are many beans and potatoes; Dr. Perlmutter specifies a bit further, recommending veggies that grow above the ground as opposed to those that grow under . . . spinach and broccoli as opposed to say, carrots and beets. Those underground vegetables, like potatoes, store sugars inside them.

It's good to cook with butter. I recently acquired some cookware to which nothing really sticks. Watch cookware demonstrations anywhere, and the sales people all say, "Oh, cook healthier, without all that fat. See the fat's dripping away from the food." Well, I like the easy clean up, but I do use butter, olive oil, and have recently discovered (and quite like!) coconut oil.

I eat plenty of cheese and dairy products, excepting, of course, ice cream. I used to eat the fruit-mixed-in yogurts, but you know what? They're as bad as ice cream, with all the added sugar. I now buy plain yogurt and blend with it *unsweetened* berries. I use whole cream in my coffee, and liberally use sour cream in many recipes. (Ok, perhaps I shouldn't have said "many" recipes; my culinary repertoire is pretty limited. But while my spectrum isn't wide, it's tasty, and being able to use these foods *while losing weight* is simply wonderful.) I do make spaghetti with either sausage or meatballs, but the pasta itself is whole grain (more fiber slows the absorption of carbs). I'll make beef stroganoff, sometimes with whole grain noodles, sometimes with rice. *Wait, isn't rice a grain, a cereal?* It is. I use brown, long grain rice. It takes longer to cook, but it's not been stripped of its fiber. I would never use a white rice, nor an instant one.

Dr. Lustig uses the phrase, "shop the outer aisles," meaning eat real foods. In virtually every supermarket, the outer aisles have the real vegetables and fruits, the real fish, the real meats, the real dairy and real eggs. And avoid anything that's been processed, anything that's in a box or a can that can sit on a shelf for weeks. If you're planning on having fish, for heaven's sake, don't buy a frozen package containing what looks like crumbs on the outside and has some "fish stuff" under that. Overall, this program and the food choices I make constitute a pretty simple plan: real foods, few carbs (and at that, those that are mostly rich in fiber), good fats and I eat until I'm full. Oh, on the subject of choices: Fresh is best, and frozen may be ok, especially if they've done nothing but flash freeze it. But avoid canned fruits and vegetables; after all the processing, there's not much nutrition left.

I eat chicken often, too. Those who hold fast to the eroding, but still prevalent conventional wisdom that red meat is bad would semi-applaud chicken as a choice. They might suggest, though, that I remove the skin. But those whom I've cited in this book, my "teachers," if you will, wouldn't agree. I'll sometimes broil chicken wings, and other times deep-fry them. When deep frying I use peanut oil.

Ultimately, if you eat like this – more or less – I'd be shocked if the weight didn't just start to fall off your frame (I can't speak to special exceptions, such as if you have a thyroid condition, or if a head injury has caused your brain to not recognize leptin (it happens)).

I used "more or less" by design. Depending on how overweight you are, or how insulin resistant you've become over your lifetime, you may not be able to have the beer. Or, you may discover you can be *less* strict than I have to be. But what's important to remember, is as your weight falls, you'll derive other benefits. Not carrying such a load may relieve your aching knees, or you may find your blood pressure returning to normal, without drugs. As Dr. Bernstein points out, some of his diabetic patients, after reducing or all-but-eliminating carbs, no longer need insulin injections.

A thought I had while writing this – remember, I'm not a scientist, and I've not bounced this off any authority – is the old adage, "Once you're a little older, your metabolism will change. It will slow down a bit and you'll gain some weight."

Ok, maybe that's all it is. Or perhaps instead, it's the fact that most of us have exposed to a moderate (or more) amount of carbs through our early lives and that as a consequence, we developed an increasing resistance to insulin. Then, sometime roughly in our mid-30's that resistance reaches a point where the increased insulin production starts the automatic turn-the-carbs-into-fat machine even though we haven't changed what we've been eating.

Which should give parents a heads-up; as well as you can, feed your kids wisely and teach them these things. Insulin resistance is gradual, building over years; fewer fiber-less carbs now pays off in later life, as the automatic-fat converter likely won't be running wide open. That's pretty clearly true, even while my own little hypothesis remains unproven.

Studies have conclusively shown that our national problem of obesity isn't because of too much food and not enough exercise. If that were the cause, Dr. Lustig asks, then why has there been a rather sudden rise in the number of obese six-month old babies? As he says, "They don't diet and they don't exercise." He answers why: believing it to be healthy (it's natural, isn't it?), mothers have given their babies apple juice.

My dad developed Alzheimer's late in his life, although it never became severe (he lived to 93, still cleared by his doctor to drive), so I have an added interest when Dr. Perlmutter, the neurologist, says that reducing carbs helps keep your brain healthy.

****

What it all boils down to is this: as a species, we didn't over the last several decades (a nano-second in evolutionary terms) suddenly mutate into gluttonous, slothful beings, incapable of controlling ourselves. The only thing that changed is what now makes up our basic foodstuff and its supply chain. Evidence of that is the rise in obesity and diabetes has globally followed industrialization and affluence. As affluence allows food to change and become more convenient, longer-lasting, sweeter and ever-more processed, obesity, diabetes and their various attendant chronic maladies rise dramatically.

Those changes to our food and supply chain didn't come about because of a sinister intent to slowly poison us, but that's been the result. When Sir Walter Raleigh introduced tobacco to Europeans, the intent wasn't to poison them, but we all know how well that turned out. And despite today knowing what we do about tobacco, we've only restricted it, not banned it. Who knows, maybe one day tobacco will be banned, but no one today has to wait to stop smoking. You don't have to wait to make these changes, either.

Reiterating one last time: the best part of all of this is achieving your weight-loss goals by eating this way really isn't hard because *there's no will power involved.* You'll eat when you're hungry and stop when you're full, not at some portion size that doesn't satisfy, or at some number of calories you calculated; you won't have to "sadly" force yourself away from the table. So not only will you avoid hunger pangs, the larger payoff is, you'll find yourself healthier, slimmer . . . *happier!*

Watch . . . listen . . . read. Remember to check with your doctor; then go *Shrink!*

LEGAL DISCLAIMER

This isn't a medical book, it is a chronicle of my personal journey through the too-common phenomenon of losing excess weight. What I've described in this book is true for me. Before beginning any dietary change or exercise regimen you should consult with your health professional.

APPENDIX

Books:

"Why We Get Fat: And What to Do About It," by Gary Taubes

ISBN: 978-0-307-27270-6c

"Fat Chance: Beating the Odds Against Sugar, Processed Food, Obesity, and Disease" by Dr. Robert Lustig

ISBN: 9781594631009

"The Great Cholesterol Myth: Why Lowering Your Cholesterol Won't Prevent Heart Disease and the Statin-Free Plan," by Drs. Stephen Sinatra and Jonny Bowden

ISBN-13: 9781592335213

"Death by Food Pyramid: How Shoddy Science, Sketchy Politics and Shady Special Interests Have Ruined Our Health," by Denise Minger

ISBN 13: 9781594631009

Websites:

The Peoples Pharmacy website:
http://www.thepeoplespharcy.com

The Diane Rehm Show's website:
http://www.drshow.org

Dr. Robert Lustig's Facebook Page:
https://www.facebook.com/DrRobertLustig

Dr. David Perlmutter's website:
http://www.drperlmutter.com/

Gary Taubes' website http://garytaubes.com/

Dr. Stephen Sinatra's website:
http://www.drsinatra.com/

Podcasts:

Gary Taubes' appearance on "The Peoples Pharmacy":

http://www.peoplespharmacy.com/2011/08/06/823-why-we-get-fat/

Dr. Robert Lustig's appearance on TPP:

http://www.peoplespharmacy.com/2011/11/26/802-sugar-hazards/

Dr. Richard Bernstein's appearance on TPP:

http://www.peoplespharmacy.com/2012/07/28/866-diabetes-dilemmas/

Dr. David Perlmutter's appearance on TPP:

http://www.peoplespharmacy.com/2013/12/14/927-how-grains-and-gluten-could-be-sapping-your-brain-power/

Transcript of Dr. Lustig's appearance on "The Diane Rehm Show":

http://thedianerehmshow.org/shows/2013-01-07/dr-robert-lustig-fat-chance-beating-odds-against-sugar-processed-food-obesity-and-0

Videos:

Dr. Lustig's "Sugar: The Bitter Truth" on youtube

http://www.youtube.com/watch?v=dBnniua6-oM

Dr. Lustig's "Fat Chance: Fructose 2.0"

http://www.youtube.com/watch?v=ceFyF9px2oY

On-line video of Dr. Stephen Sinatra & Dr. Johnny Bowden on "The Dr. Oz Show"

Part 1: http://www.doctoroz.com/videos/everything-you-know-about-cholesterol-wrong-pt-1

Part 2: http://www.doctoroz.com/videos/everything-you-know-about-cholesterol-wrong-pt-2

On-line video of Dr. David Perlmutter on "The Dr. Oz Show"

Part 1: http://www.doctoroz.com/episode/do-carbs-cause-alzheimers

Part 2: http://www.doctoroz.com/episode/do-carbs-cause-alzheimers

About the Author

Bruce Michaels says his resume resembles either "The Yellow Pages" or the lyrics to Frank Sinatra's "That's Life" (*I've been a puppet, a pauper, a pirate, a poet . . . a pawn and a king*). He has been a musician, entertainer, composer of commercial jingles, pop-songwriter, race track announcer, sports play-by-play announcer, corporate techie, operations manager for call-centers, weathercaster on television and news director for both radio and television, and TV morning-show host. He currently lives in North Carolina, where he teaches piano, performs his one-man show, "Dinner With the Rat Pack (and more!)," and is the stadium organist for the Greensboro Grasshoppers baseball club.[3]

---

[3] You can view a brief "infomercial" of his show by visiting http://www.youtube.com/watch?v=sfi8T5HP6N4 or by simply searching youtube for brucemichaelsnc .

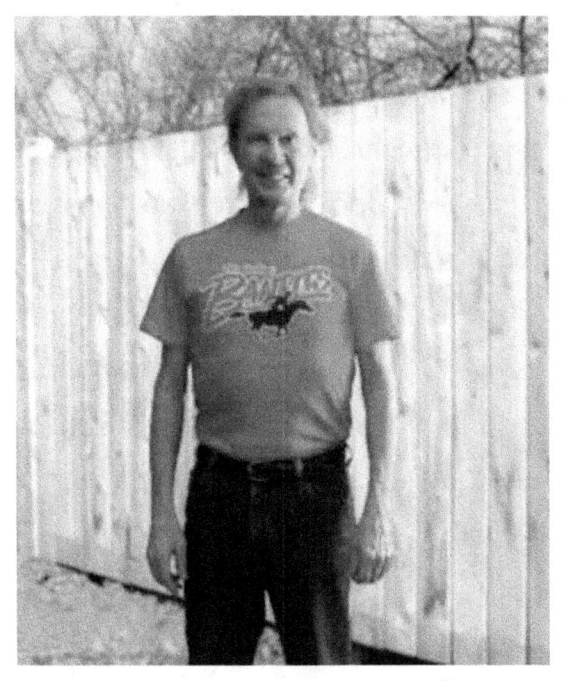

THE AUTHOR, IN FEBRUARY 2014, IN A

BOUGHT-IN-1983 T-SHIRT, BOYS' SIZE 16.

WEIGHT THAT MORNING: 111 LBS.

Contact: *bruceshrink@yahoo.com*

If you enjoyed this book, and especially if you've achieved results it, please share the news with your friends, and consider writing a review. The truths contained in this book aren't yet fully known or appreciated; were they, the obesity epidemic would no longer be an epidemic. This book surely won't change the world, but for those for whom it represents the first step in finding these truths, it can be, as all first steps are, a beginning. - b.